Holistic Therapies 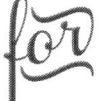 Adults with Neck Pain

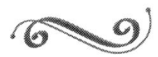

Elizabeth Meuser, PhD
Elizabeth McMaster, MSA

Copyright © 2013 Elizabeth Meuser PhD and Elizabeth McMaster MSA

All rights reserved. No part of this publication should be reproduced, stored in a retrieval system, or transmitted in form or by any means: electronic, mechanical, photocopying, recording, or otherwise, without the written permission of the autor and the publisher.)

ISBN: 1480079642
ISBN-13: 9781480079649

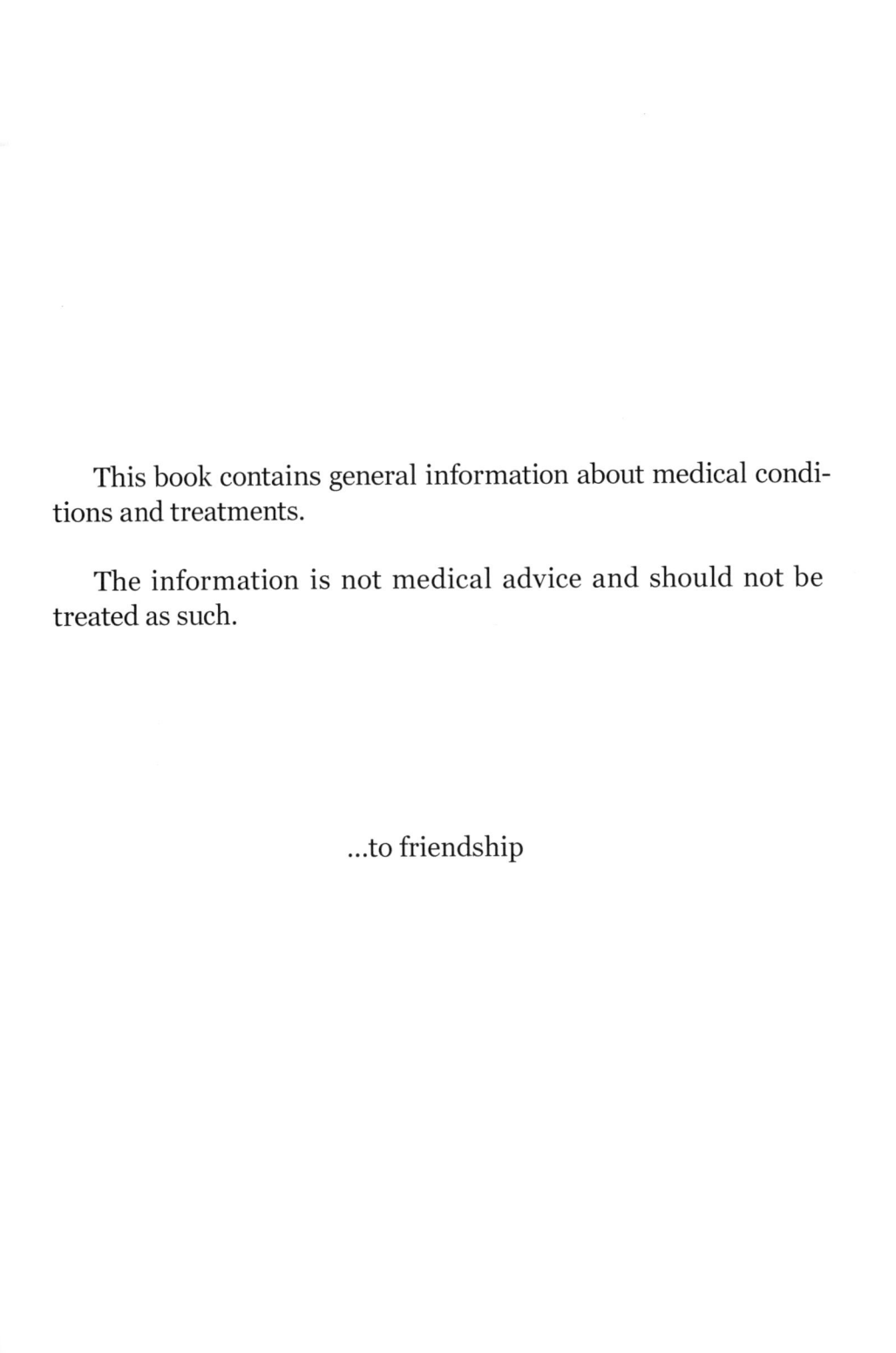

This book contains general information about medical conditions and treatments.

The information is not medical advice and should not be treated as such.

...to friendship

Table of Contents

PART ONE

Introduction — 3
About the Program — 5

Chapter One: Understanding the Basics — 9

Allopathic Medicine: The Conventional Medical Model — 10
Misconceptions about Complementary Therapies — 12
New and Necessary Ways to Think and Take Action — 13

Chapter Two: Prerequisites for Success — 15

How You Think Determines What You Get — 15
The Placebo Effect — 16
The Mind-Body Connection — 18

Intention	21
Pain: Personal Costs in Body, Mind, and Spirit	22
ALICE MCMASTER'S STORY	26

PART TWO: COMPLEMENTARY THERAPISTS AND THERAPIES

Chapter One: Introduction   29

Common Threads	29

Chapter Two: Qigong and Nutrition   37

Introduction	37
What Is Qigong?	39
What Causes Neck Soreness from a Chinese Medicine View?	41
Differences between Men and Women	43
What to Expect When You Visit a Doctor of Chinese Medicine	44
Partnering with Your Doctor of Chinese Medicine	47
Conclusion	49

Chapter Three: Chiropractic Health Care   51

Introduction	51
What Is Chiropractic Health Care?	52
What Causes Neck Soreness from a Chiropractic View?	53
Differences between Men and Women	53
What to Expect When You Visit a Chiropractor	53
Partnering with Your Chiropractor	54
Conclusion	55

Chapter Four: Acupuncture and Craniosacral Therapy   57

Introduction	57
What Is Acupuncture?	58

What Causes Neck Soreness from an Acupuncture View?	58
Differences between Men and Women	59
What to Expect When You Visit an Acupuncturist	60
Partnering with Your Acupuncturist	61
What Is Craniosacral Therapy?	63
What Causes Neck Soreness from a CST Viewpoint?	63
What You Can Expect When You Visit a CST Practitioner	64
Partnering with Your CST Practitioner	64
Conclusion	66
ALICE KASSEL'S STORY	67

Chapter Five: Natural Medicine   69

Introduction	70
What Is a Doctor of Natural Medicine?	70
What Causes Neck Soreness from a Doctor of Natural Medicine View?	71
Differences between Men and Women	73
What to Expect When You Visit a Doctor of Natural Medicine	73
Partnering with Your Doctor of Natural Medicine	74
Conclusion	75

Chapter Six: Reflexology and Bowen Therapy   77

Introduction	77
What Is a Reflexology?	79
What Causes Neck Soreness from a Reflexology and Bowen Therapy View?	80
Differences between Men and Women	81
What to Expect When You Visit a Reflexologist	82
Partnering with Your Reflexologist	83

What Is Bowen Therapy?	85
What You Can Expect When You Visit a Bowen Therapist	85
Partnering with Your Bowen Therapist	87
Conclusion	87

Chapter Seven: Yoga   89

ADELE TEDESCO'S STORY   90

Chapter Eight: Clinical Hypnotherapy and Reiki   91

Introduction	92
What Is a Clinical Hypnotherapy?	93
What Causes Neck Soreness from a Hypnotherapy View?	95
Differences between Men and Women	96
What to Expect When You Visit a Hypnotherapist	96
Partnering with Your Hypnotherapist	99
What Is Reiki?	100
Conclusion	101

Chapter Nine: Integrative Nutrition and Health Counselor   103

Introduction	104
What Is Integrative Health Counseling?	106
What Causes Neck Soreness from an Integrative Health Counseling View?	107
Differences between Men and Women	108
What You Can Expect When You Visit an Integrative Health Counselor	110
Partnering with Your Integrative Health Counselor	111
Conclusion	113

Chapter Ten: Pilates — 115

Introduction — 115
What is Pilates? — 116
What Causes Neck Soreness from a
Pilates View? — 117
What You Can Expect When You Visit
a Pilates Instructor — 119
Partnering with Your Pilates Instructor — 120
Conclusion — 123

Chapter Eleven: Physiotherapy — 125

Introduction — 126
What is Physiotherapy? — 126
What Causes Neck Soreness from a
Physiotherapy View? — 127
Differences between Men and Women — 129
What You Can Expect When You Visit
a Physiotherapist — 130
Partnering with Your Physiotherapist — 131
Ways to Manage a Painful Episode — 133
Conclusion — 135

PART THREE: PUTTING IT ALL TOGETHER

Introduction — 137
Lesson: Understand Holistic Practice — 138
Lesson: You Have Choice — 139
Lesson: Each Person's Pain Experience is
Unique — 141
Lesson: Understand the Cause(s) of
Your Neck Pain — 142
    Trauma — 142
    Poor Posture — 143
    Metabolic Changes — 143
    Poor Nutrition: Dietary Deficiencies — 144

Blocked Energy	145
Emotions	145
Self-Image	145
Stress and Challenging Relationships	146
Lesson: Pain Can Be Relieved	146
Physical Pain Relief: Medication	147
Physical Pain Relief: Posture Awareness	147
Physical Pain Relief: Exercise	148
Physical Pain Relief: Diet	148
Emotional Pain Relief	149
Social Pain Relief	149
Cognitive Pain Relief (Keeping Your Mind Active)	150
Spiritual Pain Relief	150

INDEX   153
JOURNAL WORK   157

PART ONE

Introduction

As longtime colleagues, one spring day we began a discussion about how closely our lives have paralleled over the years. Eventually our chat moved from a lazy-day conversation to a more serious consideration of the physical aspects of aging, our own and the aging of those we love. As our exchange continued, our awareness grew about the challenges chronic neck pain held for us and our circles of family and friends. So at least in part, our merging of interests for this program comes from our own aging process and from the coincidence of chronic neck pain in both of us. Even more significant, we discovered that we each have aging mothers who also share chronic neck-pain syndromes.

As we took a closer look at our mothers' individual responses, we began to notice important differences. One mother, the ninety-year-old, was and remains willing to try whatever it takes to alleviate her pain while the other, eighty-eight, prefers to "let the doctor look after it." Not unexpectedly, the ninety-year-old has been experiencing a greater quality of life than the other, who sees her neck pain as a casualty of aging.

The differing approaches of our mothers seem to mirror the architecture of our current health-care system: on one hand the system supports a conventional medical model, offering a biological mind-set that focuses on the physical body. On the other hand is a more inclusive interdisciplinary model that includes all health and health-related professionals as potential problem solvers. However, things may be changing, for there is evidence that the two practices of conventional medicine and complementary health care have been slowly moving toward a more integrated/collaborative approach. What does this mean for you? Simply stated it means you can expect an expanded circle of skilled helpers and renewed hope for a more comfortable life.

We value the collaborative view of treatment for chronic neck pain, which includes an array of diverse knowledge, skills, and mind-sets. In this collaborative approach, you, the person with the chronic neck pain, are in charge of finding solutions from a wide variety of options that best suit your unique pain experience and your chosen lifestyle. Basically, you become your own scientific experiment wherein you pick and choose any combination of therapies in order to find a solution best suited to your individual pain management needs.

We believe that when you are a true partner in your care and take part in exercising your own choice about what treatments you believe will work best for you, you will reach a better outcome. However, with you as the leader of your treatment team, progress depends on your willingness to get involved and take responsibility for the quality of your life. Getting involved means taking the time to learn about the many and varied approaches to relieve your pain and then steadily applying those approaches until you find the combination that best suits you. Our part is to help you through the maze of possibilities.

In addition to a collaborative approach, we also believe in a wellness model. A wellness model suggests that each individual has the right to perform daily tasks at his or her optimum level, regardless of ability, health challenges, or health status. Wellness can mean different degrees of health for different people but it means an improved quality of life for all. That is, even if you cannot achieve total pain relief by using a combination of approaches, at the very least, you will be able to live with an acceptable degree of discomfort. Briefly, we believe that employing a wellness model for chronic neck pain will more likely support your physical, cognitive (intellectual), social, emotional, and spiritual health in a way that allows you to be well while living with a tolerable degree of discomfort. A wellness model gives you a level of well-being that allows you to take part in whatever you choose as well as to take advantage of choices, opportunities, and activities that bring you comfort and enjoyment.

The really good news is that application of the information contained in this book will allow your body to utilize its natural response mechanisms to alleviate your pain. When your body is in balance, it can use its own intelligence to heal itself. Getting the body in balance then becomes one of the primary goals underpinning the relief and release of your chronic neck pain.

Finally, the book extends a helping hand to family members, friends, groups, and anyone on your support team, professional or nonprofessional. We believe that by expanding your knowledge and understanding about an array of approaches, you and your team will be better equipped to form the kind of partnership that can thoroughly and optimistically address your chronic neck pain.

About the Program

If life is a journey we take with others, why in my pain am I left feeling so all alone and unheard?

—Anonymous

We welcome you to a place called possibility that exists not "out there" but inside you. It is where you are healthy and whole and have all the tools you need to grow daily in your abundance of health and happiness. This health and happiness, right this very minute, are on the other side of your wall of neck pain.

The intention of this book is to help you take down the wall and lead you back to the other side. Removing the wall starts with letting go of how you traditionally thought you would reach this state of comfort and well-being. Ask yourself if it's possible that there is something you have yet to try that could be your solution? If it was not only possible but very likely, would you want to know about it?

If you answered yes to both questions, you are already on your way to healing. The "it" that is your path to a pain-free day may include one or, more likely, many new ways for treating your neck. This book shows you many options, some you may have tried, with or without success. While this book is by no means exhaustive, it will offer you a banquet of options to learn about and choose from.

No matter your age or the number of years you or your loved one has suffered, we want you to know that many people just like you have found a new path that is working for them. The path they initially took likely mirrored yours until they discovered the unique combination of therapies that was just what their body needed to move closer to a healthy and often pain-free life.

Would you like to know how?

Their stories can be found in the following pages. While each story is different, all are inspiring because of each participant's willingness to explore new avenues of healing. Moreover, every practitioner presented in the book has undertaken a self-healing journey that has only added to his or her compassion and understanding.

For example, it will be our pleasure later in the book to introduce you to Dr. Brick Saunderson, who has spent a huge part of his life as a clinical hypnotherapist. He has benefited hundreds of clients immeasurably, helping them to experience a new mastery over their symptoms. You will also meet integrative health coach Patrick Martin Jr. who found his career in complementary healthcare after having suffered his own serious health challenge.

Stand-up comedian Michael Jr. is a man blessed with the purpose of reaching out to others—often people in pain–through laughter. In a recent stand-up performance, his message was that there are "seven ways to look at every situation." Whether or not you can see in more than one way in your moments of pain, there is truth in Michael's statement. This book will give you more than one way to view your situation as well as help you understand the many possible underlying causes for your pain experience.

> *Just like the people you will meet in this book, the authors encourage you to create your own healing story and then inspire others.*

All the health-care practitioners highlighted in this book are educated in multiple ways of knowing, but they are also much more than their education. And you are much more than your pain! It is not about finding the right chiropractor, doctor of medicine, or hypnotherapist, although each may help you on your quest. We want you to be open to finding the right support for you in whatever form that may take.

Because you are reading this book, we know you are open to receiving new information, new ideas that may help you see a different way through your pain. You will not be disappointed. These pages contain the wisdom not only of alternative doctors and therapists but of fellow human beings who truly want you to experience a more pain-free life.

All are welcome; please think of us and others who have found their path as friends. If your goal is to have effective pain relief, then consider all of us part of your journey of discovery. We researched and prepared the material for this book to provide you with some options to support you on that journey.

We assume that you are reading this book because you experience neck pain more often than you would like or that you're collecting ideas for a loved one who often suffers in this way. Just for a moment, we want you to imagine what you or your loved one would do differently today if not for feeling limited by neck pain. Would you travel and visit family or friends more often? Would you get involved and help others less fortunate than yourself? Would you call someone you haven't seen in a while or invite an old friend over for tea? As you can see, there are endless ways that your life could be enriched if you or your loved one were less limited by neck pain.

Chapter One: Understanding the Basics

P ain, like your shadow companion, may tag along in everything you do. While you are awake, your discomfort may ebb and flow—sometimes bearable and other times not. Or you may experience a jarring sensation that amplifies as you move in certain directions. Emotionally, whether today is a good or bad day for you is likely linked to how much pain you are experiencing right now. Along with physical symptoms, feelings of loneliness and isolation are normal pain experiences. The aim of this book, therefore, is to restore your energy and comfort by removing the power pain has to disrupt the quality of your daily life. We want what you want—a healthier, involved, comfortable you.

But wishing without action often leads down a spiral path that ends in depression and hopelessness. We want to encourage you to remain open to the prospect that a solution is possible and that, with counsel from wise and wonderful health-care practitioners, management of chronic neck pain is within your reach, within this book. As you move through these pages and engage in the options that speak to your experience, it will become apparent that there is a healing way.

Allopathic Medicine: The Conventional Medical Model

Most of the time, most of us are able to improve our health by using solutions that have worked in the past. We know which cold remedies work best and that a cut or sore needs to be kept clean in order to avoid infection. When our own treatment plans fail, we seek the advice of our medical doctor.

Our family physicians support us by using a method called differential diagnosis to describe a specific condition. They arrive at their diagnosis through a process of investigation and elimination of multiple causes. For example, by adding and discarding possibilities for the cause of neck pain (e.g., trans mandibular joint problems, a thyroid disorder, arthritis, and spurs on the cervical spine), medical doctors can determine a primary cause. From their differential diagnosis, physicians develop a treatment plan. For some people, both cause and solution may be easily determined, and after a brief period of treatment, their problem is gone forever, never to arise again. They are considered the lucky ones.

For others, like you, pain can be more persistent. You may have found that that medication your physician has prescribed is not strong enough to take you to a place of comfort. You may be that person for whom there appears to be no end to the pain. If pharmaceuticals are the only option you have been presented with, your doctor may end up simply increasing your pain medication dosage.

Many medical doctors have a set of solutions for various conditions. For example, they may commonly prescribe a number of different pills for the treatment of chronic neck pain. Because they have had good results in the past, they assume that the prescription will help most of their patients who have similar neck pain experiences.

> *But what if—regardless of medical intervention—you continue to experience relentless pain that keeps you from fully embracing your life?*

If your pain experience has reached this point a closed mind is not your greatest asset. Rather, in this circumstance, coming from an open mind offers the critical advantage you need to manage your pain. If you remain open, you will have a much wider array of options from which to choose and, therefore, a wider range of potential solutions for relief of your neck pain. So take the time needed to answer the following questions.

What if you thought differently about using pain medication alone?

What if you confidently opened yourself up to other possible solutions?

What if your path to alleviate your pain and return to wholeness is within the realm of possibility without, or at least with a reduction in, ongoing drug therapy?

The collaborative approach that we are presenting complements the conventional medical and pharmacological approaches. If you require medication to manage your pain, you are encouraged to continue with whatever your physician has recommended. However, with the addition of complementary therapies, you may find that you require less medication to achieve the same or even better pain management.

There is no judgment here: you are the person who is the owner and operator of your body, and only you know what you want and why you make a certain choice at any given time. The contribution you bring to the table is a desire to manage your pain and a curiosity about how that is accomplished. Without desire and curiosity, your pain experience will likely remain unchanged so it will be important for you to maintain openness to new knowledge throughout your journey back to health.

Because you are the center of your personal care plan, the plan will look and feel different for each one of you. No one treatment plan will fit all neck pain experiences because every single person is unique. But with patience, each of you will find the combination of conventional and complementary treatments that will provide enhanced comfort.

Misconceptions about Complementary Therapies

Before you begin your journey, it is important to dispel any misconceptions or doubts you may have about complementary and alternative medicine. Perhaps the biggest fear is that to engage with a complementary practitioner is equivalent to being involved with someone who is not highly trained or educated. Nothing could be further from the truth. Complementary practitioners spend many years gaining knowledge and skill in their chosen field. For your interest, we have provided the academic and professional achievements of each featured practitioner in the Index at the end of the book.

Moreover, the holistic, time-intensive, and respectful way that complementary therapists work ensures that you have input into the therapy, how it is administered, and whether or not you wish to continue. Each of the therapies introduced in this book works with your body's natural ability to heal.

Another concern may be that your medical doctor would disapprove if he or she knew that you were consulting a complementary therapist. Despite the evidence, some physicians may believe that complementary medicine falls into the realm of pseudoscience; however, holistic therapy actually complements conventional/allopathic medicine. In truth, many medical doctors see the benefits gained from complementary therapies and work in tandem with holistic practitioners. Holistic practitioners are concerned with various aspects of your pain experience that include your physical, environmental, nutritional, spiritual, and emotional characteristics. Complementary and alternative therapists include client education and self-management as vital to your recovery, health, and well-being. Knowledge and self-management serve to enhance your self-confidence.

Other fallacies surround Pilates, qigong, reflexology, and acupuncture. The truth is that Pilates is not just for women; qigong is not too strenuous, nor does it take years to learn; and reflexology is more than a simple foot rub. Acupuncture actually moves one's vital energy for the purpose of balance and harmony, as do therapeutic touch, the laying on of hands, and prayer. None are sham treatments or quackery. Chinese medicine does not require a religious conversion, and, in truth, has been helping millions of people heal for over five thousand years.

In chapter two you will be introduced to some of the scientific discoveries that support holistic therapy and the reasons why you need not be apprehensive. For now, know that scientists are continually undertaking research on the effects of holistic practices. For example, we know that meditation-induced stress reduction positively supports the immune system[1] and that tai chi exercise is more effective at fall prevention in the elderly than physiotherapy.[2]

Our fears are usually based in the unknown. Therefore, before becoming involved with a therapy that is new to you, read the book and talk with others who have tried therapies outside conventional medicine. But be aware that just as science is changing conventional beliefs about the efficacy of complementary therapies, we also need to change our outdated habits of thinking and subsequent behaviors about pain and pain management. Treat your journey to awareness as a great adventure, and see how much you can learn and grow toward health and recovery.

New and Necessary Ways to Think and Take Action

Although most of us are committed to the care of those we love and want to nurture, some of us often find that there is no time to

---

[1] Contemplative Mind in Life, "Monthly Archive", *Why Mindfulness Can Help the Immune System* http://contemplativemind.wordpress.com/2012/06/ (accessed 6 Jan. 2013).

[2] Michel Tousignant, Hélène Corriveau, Pierre-Michel Roy, Johanne Desrosiers, Nicole Dubuc, and Réjean Hébert, informa healthcare, "Disability and Rehabilitation", Efficacy of supervised Tai Chi exercises versus conventional versus conventional physical therapy exercises in fall prevention for frail older adults: a randomized controlled trial, http://informahealthcare.com/doi/abs/10.3109/09638288.2012.737084 (accessed 6. Jan. 2013).

devote to ourselves in a way that respects and honors the individuals we are. For many of us, the first step down the road to our own healing is to acknowledge that we need to give the same loving care and attention to ourselves. A good place to start is with an honest self-evaluation of our habits and behaviors.

Past experiences and habits of thinking have gotten you to your current way of understanding your situation and coping with your pain. You may be one of the many with chronic pain who believe that their pain is permanent and behave accordingly. You may let pain determine your moods and actions. You may even continue to submit to a treatment that does not offer relief. Treating yourself the way you treat others—providing the same loving care—means you must treat dealing with your pain like other necessary tasks, no matter how difficult that is. Just as you learn what works for you in other areas of your life by trial and error, figuring out the best method for dealing with your neck pain requires you to try several of the options that are currently available. With persistence, you will find the combination of options presented that will provide you with your biggest reward—pain relief.

Chapter Two: Prerequisites for Success

There are many pathways that lead to healing and pain reduction. The first crucial step is to let go of the idea that your healing journey needs to look a certain way. Letting go requires you to change the way you think about your neck pain.

If you're ready to make changes in your pain experience, the way you have been managing your pain must not be working. If you continue to make the same choices, you will get the same result: continued—even worsening—pain. But living in comfort is possible if you keep an open mind, an open heart, and a belief that, with commitment and help, you will reach your destination.

How You Think Determines What You Get

We all hold powerful beliefs and expectations formed from many years of personal experience, and the way we think about our experiences forms the basis of our mind-sets. Over time our mind-set or viewpoint can become rigid. People with rigid mind-sets are usually thought of as closed-minded. In addition, they are more likely to experience pain. Their closed-mindedness causes them to develop a negative outlook that keeps them stuck in pain.

If how you think determines what you get and if you really believe that your pain cannot be managed, then you really *are* a person with unmanageable chronic pain. Others who are less rigid evaluate or think about their experiences more broadly and are thought of as open-minded. They experience less and less frequent pain. If you truly believe that there is a solution and you are open to finding it, you will master your pain. It is critical to become aware of how the way you think contributes to your pain and treatment. First, you must be willing to accept the role thought plays in embodied pain. There is scientific evidence to support how the power of your beliefs can play into your healing. Scientists call the phenomenon the *placebo effect*.

The Placebo Effect

Medical science is based on empirical evidence, which means that the treatments prescribed by medical doctors have been scientifically tested and found to be effective. The tests are supported by experiments or trials with many participants. The trials are conducted in such ways that neither the participants nor the professionals conducting the experiment know which participants are receiving the actual treatment—primarily pharmacology or surgery. For example, clients are placed into two groups; one group receives the intervention while the other is given a sugar pill, saline solution injection, or some other inert substance. Neither group is aware of which intervention it is receiving. Therefore the study is considered to be double-blind. The double-blind design is crucial because researchers can eliminate bias.

Removing bias is important because researchers can determine if the results of their study are due to the treatment, rather than to the participants' expectation of good treatment results. In science, an effect that is measurable or observable but not attributed to the prescribed treatment is called a placebo effect. In short, clients may improve despite a *sham* treatment because of their ardent belief in the effectiveness of the remedy. Their positive responses are attributed to the placebo effect.

Conventional evidence-based medicine has historically viewed the placebo effect as suspect. In other words, a placebo effect means that a client's condition is psychogenic in nature—based in a psychological rather than physiological origin. In this regard, conventional medicine considers a client's condition as arising from the mind, and, as such, exacerbated by emotional, stressful, or behavioral factors. Without supporting organic evidence, conventional medicine holds that client's only think that they're better. But; conventional medicine is rethinking its stand. Robert Burton, a medical doctor and former chief of neurology at Mount Zion-UCSF Hospital underscores the change in the medical community's thinking when he explains:

> The placebo effect has maddened the medical world for generations. But recent advances in brain imaging emphasize for me that "placebo" should not be regarded as a dirty word. In fact, it is time to give placebo a new image and update its beneficial role in our modern medical armamentarium.[3]

Recent research conducted at the National Center for Complementary and Alternative Medicine shows a physiological basis for the placebo effect that may have its origins in our genetic makeup.[4] The placebo effect can also arise outside of conscious awareness and activate the same natural brain pathways as

---

3 Robert Burton, "Why 'Placebo' is not a Dirty Word", *Salon, 1 Aug. 2008,* http://www.salon.com/2008/08/01/placebo_effect/ (accessed 4 Jan. 2012).

4 National Center for Complementary and Alternative Medicine, "Research Results-Research Spotlight", *Genetic Marker Predicts Placebo Response, a Recent Study Finds 23 Oct. 2012,* http://nccam.nih.gov/ (accessed 3 Jan. 2013).

prescribed medication.[5] The activation occurs as a result of what the intervention means to the individual. Meaning also implies that an actual medical intervention may or may not be helpful. Some individuals, who hold the belief that the treatment will not work, experience the opposite of a placebo effect—a *nocebo effect*. Again, both effects arise from individuals' thoughts and expectations, and, given accumulating scientific evidence, the medical community has been compelled to view both effects as credible. In doing so, there is a growing acceptance of holistic therapies among the medical community, and an opportunity for a more collaborative or integrated approach to healthcare.

Complementary medicine uses a holistic approach and has its origin in tradition and the importance of balance and harmony within the body's energetic system. Furthermore, complementary practitioners have long viewed the placebo effect as a positive human talent. Hypnotherapy has capitalized on the power of the mind and uses the mind's potential to help clients to self-manage pain and overcome other debilitating conditions. Moreover, the placebo effect provides support for adopting another way to think about our mind's influence on our physical health and well-being: namely, our mind-body connection.

The Mind-Body Connection

For many, many years the health-care profession treated the mind and body as two separate entities. Today, many medical professionals continue to treat either the body *or* the mind, but rarely the two as one. Recent scientific investigations have proved beyond a doubt that the body and mind do comprise one united organism that cannot be separated.

---

5 Scientific American, "Placebo Effect: A Cure in the Mind [Preview]", *In Brief,* http://www.scientificamerican.com/article.cfm?id=placebo-effect-a-cure-in-the-mind, (accessed 3 Jan. 2013)

New understandings show clearly that what affects the body is played out in the mind and what is believed or experienced emotionally affects the health of the body. Yet few of us appreciate how our thoughts affect our body, especially in terms of our personal stories. Because of the inseparable nature of human beings, many researchers now refer to us as a "bodymind." So let's take a look at how the bodymind paradox plays out.

Everyone has a story. In truth, all of us have many stories that we tell ourselves and others. These stories are important because they help to form our identity. Some stories, in particular those that are hurtful or demeaning, serve an additional purpose because they hold valuable lessons. While these lessons should be carried forward, the painful circumstances surrounding our stories need to be left behind in order for us to move ahead with our lives. Often, exceptionally traumatic experiences may stay with us for long periods of time even though we believe they have been forgotten by us. Hurtful stories tend to be carried in our bodies as well as our hearts, causing pain in both areas. To see what we mean, take a few minutes and recall a hurtful experience that you have carried with you over several years. Make your memory as vivid as possible by visualizing the circumstances as if you are in the situation now.

- *What is happening around you in your story?*
- *What do you hear?*
- *Are there scents present?*
- *Are you touching something or someone?*
- *What are you thinking in the moment?*

Many people find that recording their experiences in a journal is helpful because it enables them to get their feelings out on paper. A journal can also serve as a record of your journey so that you can look back and see how far you have come and how much you have grown spiritually and in self-awareness. You may find keeping a record of your journey through your neck pain and back to wholeness is helpful, so we have provided a few journal pages at the back of the book to get you started. The following questions begin your journal work.

As you reflected on your hurtful experience did you notice how your memory included both thoughts and feelings? Simply thinking about a painful event prompts intense emotions as if you were present now reliving the same moment.

Journal Work- Mind-Body Connection

a. Make a few notes about the circumstances surrounding your story.

b. As you recall your story, note how your body feels within the memory.

c. Is your stomach in a knot, are your teeth clenched, do your muscles feel tight? Scan your body and note where the feeling is the strongest.

d. Do you become emotional in the memory? What kind of emotion do you experience?

e. Notice the relationship between what you are thinking and what you are feeling in your memory.

What many of us fail to realize is that old hurts, slights, and fears are often at the root of our physical pain. We don't realize that the way we think and feel about past events causes pain within our bodies. People and events, past and present, can be a literal pain in the neck because the neck and shoulders are the places where tension is most commonly held.

To return yourself to harmony and peace, now complete the above exercise using the most wonderful memory you can think of. This time, recognize how your loving thoughts and feelings work together. Although we can intellectually understand the steps it takes to relieve pain, until the heart is involved in feeling and believing that pain relief is achievable, success is unlikely. We will investigate the personal costs associated with chronic pain under the heading, *Pain: Personal Costs in Body, Mind, and Spirit.*

Intention

An intention is the basis of every choice. For example, if you intend to remain centered while all around you seems chaotic, you can choose to remain quiet amid the noise and confusion. In each of your actions and thoughts, your intention is what you choose. Intention arises from consciousness, and being conscious means being self-aware.

An intention requires conscious awareness that you are actually choosing the direction of your life. In our conscious decision to share information with you, our intention is to help you make an informed choice about what you wish to do about your neck pain. Having information helps you to make a conscious choice about when to take action to relieve your neck pain and what that action will be. And a conscious, informed choice is the pathway to authentic empowerment.

To create an intention is to align your heart's desire with a goal. What you or another person may want more than anything is a life that is free from pain. Aligning this desire with a goal means that you are aligning emotion with a plan to reach that goal (e.g., intending to live more comfortably by making a choice to try two new pain management therapies over the next six to twelve months).

When heart and mind are united toward a goal and you take action, you're more likely to succeed. Success takes heart-felt belief and informed, committed action. Accomplishing your goal means that you have taken responsibility for your well-being and that self-responsibility will empower you. However, before a journey of self-discovery and self-responsibility begins, there are a few serious questions to address that may help you better appreciate how you think. The usefulness of the qualities of open-mindedness and self-honesty cannot be underestimated when embarking on a journey of self-discovery and self-responsibility. Again, we offer you some questions to move you along your journey of discovery.

Journal Work—Open-Mindedness

1. Take sixty seconds, think deeply, and record how you treat information that is new to you.

2. Do you mull it over or dismiss it out of hand?

3. Take another sixty seconds and recall a time when you simply refused to believe new information that came from a trusted source.

4. Now take another sixty seconds and recall being interested in learning new information that also came from a trusted source.

5. How did you feel in each situation?

6. How were the situations different?

7. What insights have you gained from having recalled both experiences?

How open-minded are you when new information and new situations are presented? Are you willing to not only think about but also to try new approaches to relieve your chronic neck pain?

Pain: Personal Costs in Body, Mind, and Spirit

Pain is a total-person experience that affects and is affected by the emotional, social, physical, cognitive (intellectual), and spiritual components of you. Pain produces anxiety and fear, which may make you tense, short-tempered, and reactive toward others. Irritability can drive people away, leaving you feeling misunderstood and alone.

Pain also isolates us because the physical exhaustion it produces steals our desire to engage in the world around us. It is not unusual for someone in pain to withdraw from social relationships, family, and friends. Of course, withdrawal further complicates the pain experience as depression may set in, extending periods of self-imposed isolation. A new kind of suffering is created, the kind of suffering we experience when we feel desperately alone. Lost in fear that the pain will never end, we become dispirited and despairing. Negative thoughts take over as we tell ourselves that pain is all that's left in life.

In older adults, pain can cause confusion and memory impairment, which many misinterpret as the onset of dementia. This can be both frightening and isolating. Such individuals may fear loss of independence and worry about a subsequent move from their homes to an institutional setting. Getting their pain managed is crucial for a return to mental clarity, which will in turn restore their confidence and reassure them that they can continue to live independently.

When pain is viewed as a total-person experience, medication alone is not up to the task of relieving the combination of physical, emotional, spiritual, social, and intellectual suffering. At times of penetrating loneliness, lost faith, and despair, we need a listener— someone to talk to about worries, fears, and faith—as much as we require analgesic medication.

Pain is complex, and complex problems cannot be solved with simplistic solutions. It takes a team of people—professionals, family, and friends—all working to help you find relief and comfort. Most important to team membership is you because you are the only one who can describe when, where, and the extent to which you are experiencing pain. Your care team is you-centered and you-directed. Although at the center of the team, you need not attempt to carry the burden of pain by yourself because you are surrounded by any combination of care providers available to meet your unique needs.

While you have decisional authority, you can partner with other team members to make those decisions. Partnership underscores the import role communication plays in pain management. Clear communication between you and members of your team will ensure that you receive the best pain management therapies possible.

Pain management is time-intensive because it involves testing new medications and treatments to find what combination will work best for you. Because complementary therapists work in ways that are hands-on, they have the time to listen to your concerns and encourage you throughout the process. While medical doctors in some countries are able to devote such time, in Canada, the manner in which medical doctors are reimbursed does not allow them the same luxury. In this case, collaborative health care that utilizes teamwork that values all professionals working together on your behalf proves to be a highly beneficial practice.

Care that is you-entered and directed means you have the prerogative and can choose whether or not to have recommended procedures. You are entitled to have medications and treatments explained clearly and thoroughly in a way that you understand. Some people simply put their confidence in their care providers. Other people want everything explained. Your needs may not be the same as another's; regardless, you have the right to have your needs met in a way that is acceptable to you.

True partnership requires mutual respect, collaboration, and cooperation between you and all members on your team working in your best interest. What is expected of you is that you keep an open mind and inform your care providers about how you are feeling and the degree of discomfort you are experiencing. As well, talking through your fears and concerns with your therapists and with trusted family, friends, or your spiritual advisor is recommended. As a team member, you can help yourself by increasing your water intake if needed; eating nutritional, healthy foods; and exercising to raise your mood and to keep your energy flowing. If medications are ordered, you should take them as directed in order to abate pain rather than taking them when the pain is beyond the medication's ability to alleviate it.

To demonstrate the importance of an open-minded approach and the need to involve more than one practitioner, we offer you the journey of Alice McMaster, an older woman who suffered with chronic neck pain until she found a team of health-care providers who understood her situation and worked with her to alleviate her pain.

We are grateful to Mrs. Alice McMaster for generously sharing her story and for helping others with neck pain to remain hopeful and find comfort.

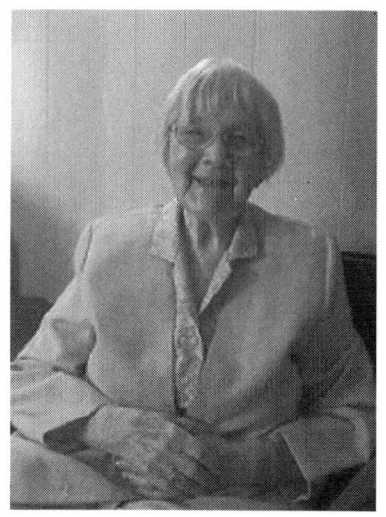

ALICE MCMASTER'S STORY

The following was graciously provided by Elaine Cameron, daughter of a brave woman, Mrs. Alice McMaster, who is the center of the story. Mrs. McMaster epitomizes our reason for writing this book. She is an exemplar for any older adult suffering with neck pain. At eighty-nine years old, Mrs. McMaster began her journey to discover collaborative therapies that could help relieve her very serious neck condition. At her advanced age, she remained open-minded and willing to sift through a variety of complementary therapies to decide on those that she believed would be helpful to her. She was also mindful to follow through on the treatment advice and guidance provided to her by her network of practitioners. At ninety-one, her days are a rich tapestry of family and friends as she is again able to fully engage in her life. This is her story, told by her daughter:

My mother, Alice McMaster, is now ninety-one years old. Sometimes I forget that fact. Others do, too. Many people who know my mother will comment on her progressive views, her sympathetic understanding of others, and her zest for continued learning.

In the last couple of years, she has had to contend with cervical radiculopathy, a real pain in the neck. Very real! At its worst she could not dare to move her head even slightly, or she would feel the jolting pain of the pinching of a nerve. She wore a neck brace, she did not drive in cars, and she took a great deal of Tylenol.

Today, many months after her original diagnosis, her neck is again mobile; her pain, at its very worst, is a mere two out of ten. This is the story of how this recovery came to be, how a ninety-one-year-old found the help she needed and got better.

"The main thing I had going for me was I had a good doctor," my mother answered when I asked what she felt was the most significant factor in her recovery. "What did he do?" I asked. "Well, he took me himself to the physiotherapist, and he said to her, 'What can you do for this lady?' And he referred me to an arthritis specialist!"

What my mother did not say, but what I believe is the underlying message of her doctor's actions, was, "It does not matter your age. We are going to help you deal with your condition and do whatever can be done to make it better."

So she started with the physiotherapist, who gradually, carefully helped Mom gain small fragments of movement. She gave her a neck brace, which she wore when needed. It helped, too. The arthritis specialist prescribed Pennsaid and Pennsaid rub.

After many months, she also was included in a pain clinic where a group of specialists helped her and others by introducing them to coping strategies to reduce long-term pain. They also provided encouragement and helped my mother lessen the amount of Tylenol she was taking.

But there were other things that helped in her recovery. She itemized these: "I had a small, curved pillow. And with it, I never had a problem sleeping. Also, in the last six months, I have started doing exercises." My sister Patricia who had taken lessons in qigong taught this very gentle form of exercise to my mother and father. "It helps." My mother, never one to find time for exercise before, concedes with a small smile. "Also, I am lucky I don't have a lot of commitments, so I can rest when I need to, and that helps."

Knowing that my mother has taken nutritional supplements for years, I asked about this. "Well, a few years ago, I stopped taking them for a while, and I found I tired more easily during that time, so I started taking them again and have never stopped since."

With that, she got up from the table to put on the kettle. She looked back toward me and smiled. "You just have to keep rolling along, I guess."

You, too, can find your mix of solutions toward getting back to doing the things you love to do. Perseverance helps; encouragement helps, too. Cervical radiculopathy can be beat. Someday you will be able to look back with a smile yourself.

Alice McMaster is only one person who has been helped by the choices that she, with the support of her family, has made to find her way through pain and back to health. There are many, many stories like hers; stories of people willing to try complementary health strategies and have realized an improved quality of life. You can be one of them.

PART TWO: Complementary Therapists and Therapies

Chapter One: Introduction

In part two, you will be introduced to an array of health-care providers. These practitioners provide therapies and treatments that complement the work of your medical doctor. Your medical doctor is a member of your health-care team as are other complementary practitioners you may choose to seek out for help.

Common Threads

During the exploration and interview processes for the development of this book, we were struck by the similarities among these complementary practitioners' personal stories. Without exception, all of the practitioners you are about to meet feel that the work they are undertaking to assist people back to health and well-being is a call to service. One therapist spoke of being "divinely guided" throughout her training and her career in complementary medicine.

Many spoke to us of their own difficult journeys and how in becoming more self-aware and spiritually present, they overcame challenges while simultaneously pledging their commitment to others who were in some way hurting. Their compassion for their fellow human beings is palpable.

All of the practitioners emphasize a holistic approach: that is, they practice in such a way that they attend to the physical, emotional, cognitive, social, and spiritual needs of each individual. Few of the practitioners we interviewed are limited to only one way to help their clients. Most are schooled in multiple treatment modalities so that their approach to treatment really does address the total client.

Most of these practitioners' therapies involve hands-on treatments in an environment where touch is continuous and, as a result, reaching the heart of another is more easily achieved. They often mention the joy that they find in their work and how working in partnership gives them a valued opportunity to keep learning about the application of remedies and also about themselves. We know that their wisdom will help you to learn and grow despite your physical discomfort and suffering.

One important consideration as you begin your journey toward self-healing is that not all people are the same. It is of utmost importance that you and your therapist are a good match. A partnership is like a bird; if a bird is trying to fly with only one wing, it cannot succeed. In other words, if you find that you and the practitioner you have initially chosen are not communicating effectively, find another. You need not work with someone if you feel that your needs are not being met. And; because people are so different, be aware as well that your practitioner may find it difficult to work with you and suggest that you find another. One of the reasons for miscommunication may be that you and your practitioner differ in the goals that you have for yourself. Or, there may be a misunderstanding in how much discomfort you are experiencing compared with your therapists' impression. On-going communication is essential within effective partnerships.

We begin part two by offering you the wisdom that underscores the rest of this book, knowing that you will greatly appreciate the words of Dr. Brick Saunderson,

The question has often been asked of me over the years as a therapist, "How do you understand human suffering?" What we do know is that, as humans, we are very complex. Over the centuries Western culture has taken on what is known as rational or "Greek" thinking. What this means is that we have compartmentalized everything. This of course is very evident in health care. When we are suffering physically, we go to our medical health provider (doctor, chiropractor, or physiotherapist).

When we suffer emotionally, we go to a mental health provider (psychologist or counselor). When we suffer spiritually, we go to a minister (priest, rabbi, shaman, or advisor). We have neatly divided ourselves up into parts. But maybe we need to rethink this. We need to think of ourselves as a whole—not just a body, nor just a mind, nor just a spirit, but a complete interconnected being: soma-psyche-pneuma.

As holistic therapists, often when we explore disease in a person, we focus on emotions and how they manifest physically in the body or body syndromes and how they relate to the emotions. Just as often, we bypass that third essential part of the whole: the spirit, the key to healing.

Wayne Dyer has pointed out, and rightly so, that we are all spiritual beings having a human experience. What does this mean? How is it connected to wellness and wholeness in one's journey? The fact that we are spiritual beings having a human experience is a profound truth. This truth is universal in the human experience. No matter where you go you find that all humanity is drawn toward a higher, greater other. The simple premise that we are spiritual beings attests to this fact. I am not speaking of religion or dogma, per se, but rather the reality of knowledge that if we exist, then something greater than us must also exist. We find this built into human DNA. No matter where human experience is found, you find the need to connect with this greater other in order to find meaning for existence.

Why is the inclusion of the spiritual part of a person so important to the healing journey? Because it is the connection of our spiritual being to the greater other that gives us hope. It is the very idea that we are not alone, that we are connected to this other, greater than us alone, that anchors us to the possibility that our suffering is not in vain. It gives meaning to our existence and strength to draw on to be overcomers.

Like Dr. Saunderson, the practitioners you are about to meet represent some of the best in their field. Their individual therapies, although equally important are presented in no particular order. We have also used the pronouns *he* and *she* interchangeably to avoid the use of discriminatory language.

Each Practitioner's contribution is formatted in the same way beginning with a brief description of his or her personal journey toward a career in complementary healthcare. Next, each therapist provides a description of his or her field of practice followed by an examination of the underlying causes for neck pain according to his or her discipline. The information is intended to educate and enlighten. Differences between men and women from each practitioner's lived experience are provided because often these differences are overlooked.

Recognizing that new experiences can provoke anxiety, we spend time outlining what you can expect when you visit a complementary practitioner according to each therapist's treatment strategy. Because partnership is all important in the success of your therapy, we offer ways to work effectively in partnership with your therapist. However, these are only rudimentary and will be discussed with you at the time of your treatment and the development of your personal treatment plan. We sincerely hope that the formatting is informative and will assist you in making a decision to consult with a complementary/alternative health practitioner.

To honor the educational background that informs each therapist's practice, we have included an index at the back of the book. In this way, you will understand the hard work and commitment required by these incredible professionals who dedicate their lives daily to people just like you. All therapists are registered and/or certified by their professional organizations.

It is no small accomplishment to spend one's life in service to his or her fellow humans. We have been blessed to have worked with each of them.

We invite you to learn and enjoy!

Chapter Two: Qigong and Nutrition

Laraine Crampton is a practitioner of Chinese medicine in private practice at Healing Life Traditional Chinese Medicine in Santa Monica, California. She is an accomplished acupuncturist and has developed a lifetime practice in qigong. The following quotes were provided by Laraine on August 21, 2012. We thank Laraine for her contribution to the section on qigong and nutrition.

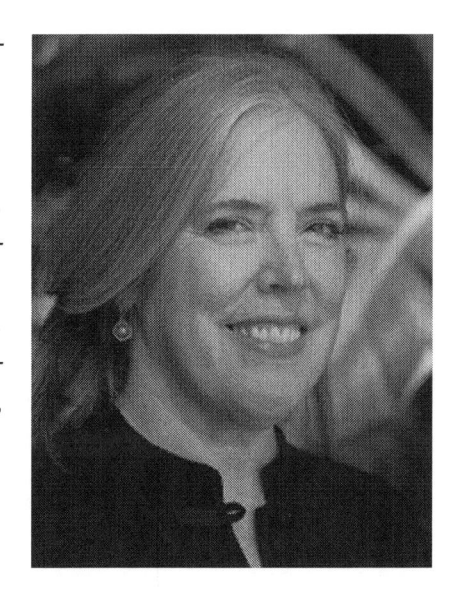

Introduction

The recognition of the self as healer often begins with one's own healing. In the late eighties and early nineties, Laraine found herself in a health crisis. At the time, her alarming symptoms fit no recognized medical diagnosis. Her story will be familiar to many who have experienced being unwell but unable to determine exactly why. Laraine recalls her own experience, "Many medical doctors I consulted said that they could not do anything. They would say, 'Well, there's something wrong with you, but we don't know what it is.' Or, 'there's nothing wrong with you; it's all in your head.'"

Her symptoms were finally understood in part as chronic fatigue syndrome. The Centers for Disease Control calls it a "debilitating and complex disorder" that affects many body systems and includes symptoms of weakness, muscle pain, problems with memory and concentration, and an inability to receive restorative sleep. [6] Such symptoms can be frightening. This was especially the case for Laraine because, at the time of her illness, the medical community knew little about CFS and had little to offer in the way of treatment. Today CFS is better understood and treated in both allopathic and complementary ways. Fortunately, a friend suggested to Laraine that she try acupuncture. At first, Laraine was as afraid of the treatment as she had been of the symptoms.

> I'm a little embarrassed to admit this, but it's true. I was terrified of acupuncture because I knew nothing about it or the culture behind it. I was afraid that I would end up in a strange office with someone pushing needles in me, not knowing what was happening or what to do. It took me three months to gain the courage to consult with my friend's acupuncturist. When I finally did, of course, I realized that my fears were the natural fear of the unknown, and they dissolved.

One of the most helpful approaches that Laraine's acupuncturist offered was to instill great confidence that acupuncture—along with Chinese medicine and improved nutrition—would restore

---

[6] Centers for Disease Control and Prevention, "Chronic Fatigue Syndrome," http://www.cdc.gov/cfs/ (accessed 9 Sept. 2012).

Laraine's body's vital energy and lead to her successful recovery within a short period of time. He encouraged her to monitor her own progress by way of diet and exercises that she could manage by herself. However, Laraine was not entirely comfortable with the treatment. She explains:

> Again the fear factor showed up, and it took me a few weeks to get past my anxiety about these exercises that were dealing with my "life energy." The idea was very foreign to me. I had grown up knowing that I had bones and blood and that sort of thing, but the notion of messing with my vital energy seemed foreign and frightening. I worried that it might be in conflict with my faith and that I would have to give up either qigong or my faith in order to get well.

Laraine was to learn there was no conflict with or need to forfeit her faith. Qigong meant working with her breath, gentle exercise, and her body's qi (energy) to make positive changes in her overall health. She continues to practice qigong and eat in ways that support and sustain her body.

Laraine's experience with her acupuncturist convinced her that she wanted to help others as she had been helped. She learned qigong and practiced her training for a few years before moving on to study acupuncture and Chinese medicine. She recalls learning that the system of Chinese medicine looks to the seasons to understand how our diet and health are affected by seasonal energies such as heat and cold. Like the seasons, foods have energetic properties that are warm, cold, invigorating or calming. Even if the energy is subtle, it can have an influence on health.

In addition to acupuncture, Laraine's training in Chinese medicine incorporated nutritional therapy, herbal medicine, a body therapy similar to massage, and the practice of qigong. The curriculum at her particular school required extensive training in qigong throughout the intensive four years of her degree work.

What Is Qigong?

Qigong is a Chinese practice of healing and energy medicine that uses a wide array of exercises, both formal and informal, many of which are ancient, handed down through family lineages over 2,500 years of Chinese history. Other qigong exercises are more contemporary. Whether following the traditional or contemporary methods, with a bit of training and coaching, almost anyone can practice qigong. It may resemble tai chi, or yoga; it may be as simple as walking, sitting, or reclining in quiet and purposeful focus. Laraine outlines the practice:

> Qigong asks the person practicing it to use her attention, to incorporate her breath, and to also make some intention in harmony with movement. One of the key things qigong does is to bring oxygen and blood flow to the whole body and whichever specific area the individual wants to focus on. The movements of qigong—in other words, the "efforts" of qigong—are gentle; they're often slow, usually calm movements, and more often subtle.

The essence of qigong is holistic. It addresses the spiritual aspect in that it is all about engaging the body, the breath, the mind, and the spirit to bring more oxygen and vital energy to the body and specifically to the areas that the individual intends to heal. In this way, it provides a sense of connection, coherence, wholeness, and vitality to the individual.

When used for neck pain, stiffness, and discomfort, qigong helps with relaxation by opening the shoulders and the neck in central ways. It reunites neck and shoulder functioning with the rest of the body. This helps to restore circulation and freedom of movement very gently and gradually as the client is quietly breathing and moving; attending to the whole body along with the area he wishes to heal. Laraine demonstrates this notion:

One of my patients calls it her Macarena. I find it charming that she talks about qigong that way. When she raises her arms over her head and relaxes her neck, back, shoulders, and arms as she breathes and pays attention in her self-styled dance, she is practicing qigong as much as anyone performing the formal exercises.

What Causes Neck Soreness from a Chinese Medicine View?

Laraine outlines three things that underscore neck discomfort and pain in older adults—a person's history of accident or injury, levels of daily activity, and the overall health of the spine from the neck to the lower back.

Neck injury through falls, motor vehicle accidents, or postural strain can have a profound effect as we age. The long-term effects can be compounded if such injuries have been dismissed as nothing serious, and consequently, left untreated at the time of initial injury. In truth, we sometimes forget about injuries, especially if they happen at a time when we have other things on our minds. An incident that may be dismissed as "a little whiplash" can later cause serious discomfort and pain. Laraine mentions several such client responses:

> When I ask clients, "Have you ever had a serious injury of the neck?" they'll say no. And then sometime later, sometimes several visits later, they will volunteer the fact that they were in a serious automobile accident when they were twenty, and then another one when they were thirty-five, and then again at fifty. But no problem—all they had was a little whiplash.

Jarring the neck when inattentive and busy with other activities is another injury that can go unnoticed. Laraine gives an example:

> A young mom carrying her child while lifting heavy bags, trying to navigate stairs while she's trying to manage the child and carry groceries may hurt her neck and think nothing of it because she's got to go on to the next thing. She may deal with a little neck pain for a few days but may not think anything of it. ...Five to ten or fifteen years later, that little tweak may have grown to some limitation of movement or accumulation of the effects of that brief and forgotten injury. Over time, it's those kinds of things that cause problems.

Doctors of Chinese medicine also consider how an individual's daily activities can contribute to pain and discomfort in later years. Desk work, hobbies, and simply sitting for long periods all put us at risk for neck problems. Seniors who spend time with newer technologies such as computer searches, e-mail, and texting friends may find that these activities contribute to neck pain. All activities requiring that the head and neck be held in one position for an extended time are counter to what human beings need for neck strength and comfort. Laraine explains:

> Most of us as children would be freely looking in every direction, looking to the side, over our shoulder, turning our heads to see what the world looks like backward or upside down. So that natural impulse is to keep our whole body moving freely and in multiple directions as we needed to do in human history, climbing into trees and caves and up hills while keeping an eye on our environment. So when we limit ourselves to sitting in one place and staring in one direction, it causes the muscles to tire very quickly and get very restless, and that can lead to early signs of pain...activity levels are very important in accumulating pain as well as relieving it.

The third area for consideration is the overall health of the spine. Chinese medicine addresses many of the postures, movements, nutrients, and so forth that determine the health of the spine. One of the most important considerations is the degree of movement or impairment of movement in our lower backs as we age. Laraine advises that if the back isn't moving and the lower back isn't healthy, then the neck is going to try extra hard to compensate for the lack of movement, and so you have a neck that works even harder and gets more tired as it fights to compensate for an immovable back.

Differences between Men and Women

Although the practitioner sees each client as a unique individual, Laraine has noticed some general differences between men and women in how they respond to a painful experience. Women, throughout their adult lives, have had to be keen observers on behalf of their children and families as well as for their own safety. They tend to be the care providers whose job it is to notice what others are experiencing so that they can provide support and comfort. Being other-centered may mean that they are less inclined to pay attention to their own comfort.

When older women are in the throes of a painful and long-standing neck and shoulder condition, it seems that they're comparing their current weakened state to the women they once were—and falling short. Not used to being the one requiring support and attention, older female clients present different challenges. Here's what Laraine has encountered:

> Older women seem at times to take things more personally and can be more saddened or more hurt or upset by pain. Sometimes it seems an indicator of personal defeat. You know: I tried to get over this but I just can't. They hold themselves to a higher standard of deserving and asking for help. So sometimes with older women, I am not only treating the physical problem, but I am also comforting them about feelings they have about chronic pain.

Older men differ in that they want to be seen as strong and present themselves as able to manage whatever age has in store for them. Just as they ignored and overcame the discomfort of hard contact sports in their early years, they expect to do so with any discomfort that comes along as they grow older. Laraine explains, "The challenge is to have them take their pain seriously so that they can do something about it rather than see it as something they just have to live with." Gender differences are important in how a doctor of Chinese medicine evaluates and treats neck pain.

What to Expect When You Visit a Doctor of Chinese Medicine

When you visit a doctor of Chinese medicine, expect to have a complete assessment and to provide a health history. Although we are discussing qigong and nutrition in this section, doctors of Chinese medicine use many other tools to work toward the restoration of your health and well-being.

Not only are they interested in restoration of health, but they also work to prevent problems from occurring in the first place. Laraine provides two examples:

> I have a carpenter, fifty-two years old, who recognizes that the joint problems that come from excessive hammering now will still be there at sixty-two and eighty-two. Helping him to find healthy ways to reduce inflammation and poor circulation is important now to promote a balanced and healthy life so he can retire and enjoy other things...helping young adults to discover a healthy diet so they don't have at sixty or eighty to suddenly have to undo all the damage of a lifetime of poor diet.

Laraine believes in taking responsibility for one's own health regardless of one's age or presenting problem. Laraine encourages all of her clients—even those in later years, at seventy, eighty, or ninety—to learn what they can do for themselves rather than spend their retirement funds on continual physician visits and prolonged dependence on pharmaceutical products. She coaches her clients toward healthier lifestyles. It is her practice to consider, lifestyle changes in diet, portion sizes and nutrient allowances, and daily exercise including incorporating walking, breathing/ mindfulness of breath. She is careful to consider "not just what kind of treatment [she] can offer but also what [her clients] can do."

Doctors of Chinese medicine believe that two of the most important habits that you can adopt are qigong and healthy dietary changes. Introductory qigong may be as simple as learning to relax in a standing, sitting, or lying position and using gentle breathing and movement. As you become more accomplished with breathing and intention, you may be introduced to yoga-like or tai chi exercises.

Your doctor of Chinese medicine will help you to become more conscious of your posture in walking habits, sitting and rising positions, and managing stairs. Often, older adults develop habits such as stooping over to walk down stairs or staring at and shuffling their feet as they walk. For safety, each of these habits needs correction so that the neck, shoulders, and back are in the appropriate upright position for healthy balance as well as to prevent strain and potential falls.

Nutrition is a major area in Chinese medicine that is also addressed in restorative care for the neck. When the tendons, ligaments, and arteries of the neck have grown stiff or inflexible, it is important to ensure that one's diet includes adequate nutrients, oils, and essential minerals to restore flexibility and adaptable tissues. "It is also helpful," Laraine adds, "to use a scarf or shawl around the neck for protection from the cold to keep structures flexible and adaptable."

Laraine continues the discussion on the importance of choosing foods with high nutrient value when she claims:

> One of the things that we contend with as we reach middle age and beyond is that we see results of "you

are what you eat." As we grow older, the body begins to deliver the consequences of what we have been eating every day for all of our lives...some of us have developed habits that every morning of our lives, instead of a nutritious breakfast, we've had a only piece of toast and a cup of coffee or some other dietary habit that has been ingrained and that may eventually not serve us very well.

One of the main conditions that older adults develop that causes neck pain, stiffness, and inflexibility is osteoarthritis. Bone spurs from the accumulation of calcium and poor circulation may also accompany the inflammatory condition. Diet can play a critical role in reducing the potential for bone spurs, managing an appropriate amount of calcium to maintain bone, and helping to restore flexibility in the neck. Laraine refers to findings on the effect of wheat proteins on calcium management. "If older people are eating wheat on a daily basis in crackers, bread, pastries, and pastas, they are more likely to develop inappropriate accumulations of bone including the development of bone spurs." warns Laraine.

Therefore, if you are experiencing neck and shoulder pain, one of the things that may be recommended by your practitioner of Chinese medicine is to reduce or eliminate wheat and wheat-based products. Thankfully, there are many other grains from which to choose. For example, quinoa is a grain from South America that can be eaten as a breakfast food or added to salads. Many specialty bakers are now using non wheat grains such as millet, oats, and quinoa.

Whether or not you are gluten sensitive, adopting a gluten-free diet can prove to be a healthy choice while offering diversity in your choices. Laraine thinks that "it's wonderful to change things up, and eating a gluten-free cookie or muffin can be a lovely change whether you're sensitive to gluten or not."

Sugar contributes to inflammation, and a steady input of sugar in the body feeds inflammation. Inflammation causes swelling and pain and compromises circulation. Therefore, it is better to get sweetness from natural sources such as fruit and honey. Unrefined honey is particularly advantageous because it contains enzymes that help to reduce inflammation.

Chinese medicine aims to return the body to its natural balanced state so being conscious of sugar and salt intake is another important factor when changing to a healthier diet. Laraine notes the impact of aging taste buds on diet when she explains:

> As we spend more years on this planet our taste buds and sense of taste can gradually be eroded or diminished to some degree, and we begin to want more flavor—sweeter sweets, saltier salts, more peppery peppers. One consequence of this is that sneaking a little sweet after a meal or deciding to have a bowl of ice-cream in the evening can actually work against us in quite significant ways. Sugar is one of life's foods for all kinds of organisms, including pathogens such as yeast, bacteria, and viruses that love to be fed by our sugar uptake and take up real estate in our bodies.

Laraine also cautions against the use of artificial sweeteners as the unintended consequence of putting artificial sweeteners into the marketplace is that products containing artificial sugar create a craving for more sweet-flavored foods and more sugar to satisfy the craving. To combat the situation, Laraine advises that her patients, "head straight for naturally sweet fruit...take a break, even for a week or two, from artificially sweetened sugars and then eat a ripe blackberry or fresh blueberry and see how amazing it tastes. There's a lot of natural sweetness to it." You may be surprised to find that foods considered to be bland have a subtle flavor once sugar has been eliminated. Making dietary changes can seem difficult at first, but, by taking small steps over a few weeks or months, can help you reach your goal of a more pain free life.

Partnering with Your Doctor of Chinese Medicine

Whenever we are provided with new information and new interventions to restore health, we are challenged by our commitment to follow through. It is not easy but taking responsibility for our own health and well-being can make the difference between having no hope and having optimism for a better future. The choice is always ours.

When partnering with your doctor of Chinese medicine, a practice that will be very helpful to adopt is a walking routine. Recall that practicing qigong can be as simple as walking, especially when combined with mindful breathing. Walking is a wonderful way to relieve the tension that we carry in our spines, shoulders and neck. Many health-care professionals believe that walking is the optimal exercise for our backs, necks, and shoulders. Walking also improves cognition—our brain function—by increasing oxygen flow, which has the happy outcome of improving memory and concentration. Walking also stimulates the production of endorphins, the brain's natural pain relievers, and lifts feelings of depression. Increasing activity and movement can be fun, and the health benefits are certainly worth it.

Chinese medicine encourages hydration to help the body's cells communicate, which in turn keeps our brains active and alert. Increasing fluid intake offers other benefits such as maintaining the ability of intervertebral cushions to relieve stress on spinal nerves and bones. The chance of a bladder infection is significantly reduced, inflammatory wastes are cleared, skin tone improves, and the by-products of stress are discarded via urine. Some people drink too much fluid and others too little. The challenge is to drink adequate amounts without overdoing it. Laraine provides the following advice:

> Recognize that each eight ounce glass of water or liquid is part of your portion for the day and you only need about eight to ten of those glasses a day, whether that's a cup of soup, cup of tea, or glass of water. Getting those

evenly distributed throughout the day is getting our brains hydrated and helps our urinary tract to manage its challenges.

Additional activities that you, as partner, can perform include completing your daily exercise program as prescribed, eating healthy snacks, conforming to recommended dietary changes, and getting adequate rest. Comfort measures that you find helpful such as the use of bean bags and soft collars are to be used in moderation and primarily if you are reclining in a chair or lying in bed. It is advised that soft collars be used only in an acute inflammatory period because using them on a regular basis will actually weaken your neck muscles and will eventually cause additional problems with pain and stiffness.

Because Chinese medicine takes a holistic approach, it is important to mention the psychological basis for neck and shoulder pain. Women tend to be more open to a psychosocial, emotional, and spiritual probe into physical health issues. Laraine provides an explanation of the interplay among these critical factors.

> If there is stiffness, I'll gently ask my patients what they're being stubborn about in their lives or where they're being rigid in their approach to others. When I've asked, "Where are you rigid in your life, where are you stiff, what fears or critical attitudes do you hold?" I've often seen them breaking down in tears and heard, "Well I've been angry with my son for thirty-five years," or, "My daughter-in-law doesn't keep house the way I think she should, and I just can't stand to be in her house; it hurts every time I go there." When we begin to realize that our attitudes toward ourselves or others are stiff or rigid, then we can begin to relax those attitudes. Then, voila, the neck and shoulders begin to relax.

These are important insights, and part of partnering to restore health involves self-reflection and self-honesty. Only when we begin to become aware of old patterns of thought and action are we able to break through those patterns in our journey to health and well-being. Changes such as those mentioned are best made in partnership. Your doctor of Chinese medicine works with you to accompany and encourage you along a new path toward your goal of a pain free life.

Conclusion

Chinese medicine with its emphasis on qigong and healthy nutrition can play an important role in helping you to regain your power over what may feel like an insurmountable condition marked by constant pain, discomfort, and stiffness. The gentle exercises, breathing, and concentrated intention combined with healthy whole foods prescribed by your doctor of Chinese medicine can offer comfort and relief. Avoiding sugar and other dietary triggers serves to reduce inflammation and also eases pain and discomfort and reinstates hope for recovery. All these rewards are possible from your willingness to try a holistic approach in partnership with your doctor of Chinese medicine.

Chapter Three: Chiropractic Health Care

Dr. David WU is a doctor of chiropractic and clinical nutritionist located in Diamond Bar, California.

The following quotes are from a May 17, 2012 interview with Dr. Wu. We thank Dr. Wu for his contribution to the following section on chiropractic health care.

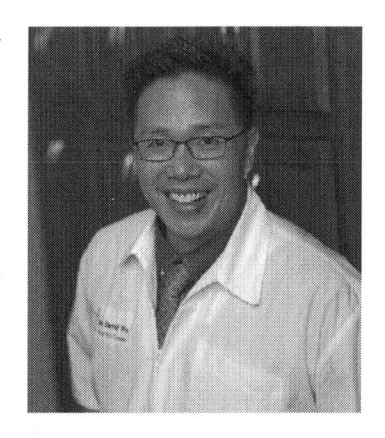

Introduction

Dr. David Wu's choice to become a doctor of chiropractic was not a career selection any of his fellow school mates would have guessed was his calling. He is a self-confessed former sugar-holic. His book *Confessions of a Sugar-Holic: A Journey to Health and Rediscovery* chronicles his addiction to and recovery from an eating habit high in processed sugar and the lessons he learned on his way back to health.

Now a highly sought-after holistic healer, Dr. Wu recognizes that nutritious foods, spiritual practice, and the application of sound chiropractic principles guide the quality of his life and the care he provides. As he listens to and treats his clients, he also educates them so that they know how they can begin to address the underlying causes of their neck pain and the lifestyle changes that will help them heal.

What Is Chiropractic Health Care?

Chiropractic has been around for more than one hundred years because it is such a helpful treatment for people who have health challenges including back and neck pain. Doctors of chiropractic believe that health challenges arise from the spine and the nerves that are housed by and extend from the spine. They use a noninvasive, hands-on approach for people who are experiencing difficulties related to their spine, nervous system, pelvis, and joints.[7]

Chiropractors provide diagnosis, treatment, and preventive care for the total person. Providing care for the whole person means approaching every person with the understanding that each is an individual with his or her own unique physical, emotional, cognitive, and spiritual makeup. Basically, chiropractors address the complex nature of these interacting components of human beings through structural (physical) adjustment, emotional support (how you feel about your discomfort), cognitive reframing (how you think about your discomfort), and spiritual awareness (how you live with pain).

---

[7] Ontario Chiropractic Association, "Chiropractic Care", *What is Chiropractic?* http://www.chiropractic.on.ca/chiropracticcare/whatischiropractic.aspx (accessed 12 May 2012).

What Causes Neck Soreness from a Chiropractic View?

Adults who attribute neck discomfort to aging may assume that the pain is due to the natural development of arthritis that gets worse over time. But similar descriptions of neck pain in two different people can have unique causes. Dr. Wu notes that he pays attention to the internal organs of each person because he knows that neck pain can also be the result of liver and digestive problems. Like Dr. Wu, all chiropractors use a combination of treatments, all of which are grounded in their client's specific needs and based on their client's description of neck pain.

Differences between Men and Women

There are some differences to consider between genders. For example, aging women in many cases tend to experience heavier demands on their health than do aging men. Although neck pain can be a problem for both men and women, Dr. Wu sees a higher number of female clients. One reason for this is hormonal changes and their effect on the spine and joints in women. Things like weight gain and depression, common in pre- and postmenopausal women, can be an underlying cause of chronic neck pain.

By understanding the role that aging plays in chronic neck pain, you can begin to understand how your emotions also contribute to your experience of pain. Emotional changes are changes in the body's interior chemistry related to diet, hormones, medications, and individual responses to pain, especially long-standing or chronic pain.

What You Can Expect When You Visit a Chiropractor

You will be asked to give the chiropractor your complete medical history so that he can make a comprehensive diagnosis and treatment plan. He will recommend beneficial exercises and other noninvasive therapies such as spinal adjustment for realignment. Many of the suggestions that your chiropractor will have will relate to lifestyle changes. Lifestyle counseling is a component of good chiropractic care and includes discussion about changes in nutrition, diet, and activity with recommendations for each. Depending on the assessment, your chiropractor may also choose to refer you to another specialized practitioner to help you make successful lifestyle choices.

Your chiropractor is interested in the "total" you, so expect him to ask questions concerning your medication. Some anti-inflammatory medications for pain such as ibuprofen can cause high blood pressure and tax your liver and kidneys when used long-term. If you are living with chronic neck pain, you likely have been taking some form of anti-inflammatory medication. If your pain can be managed to the point where it no longer interferes with daily living, then being able to reduce or to stop taking these medications is beneficial for your overall health and well-being.

Chiropractic treatment usually requires a few visits. Whether your pain is acute or chronic, treatment continues until you and your chiropractor determine that you are improved. Often, after a break from treatment, it is necessary to resume for a period of time. Because of the chronic nature of neck pain, it is vital to your recovery that you are willing to follow through on and participate in your treatment plan.

Partnering with Your Chiropractor

You probably remember the discussion from chapter one, Pain: Personal Costs in Body, Mind, and Spirit, where the consequences of unrelieved neck pain are outlined. As a result, you are aware that chronic pain can leave a person feeling helpless and hopeless: helpless because what has been tried so far has not been successful and hopeless because of a belief that nothing more can be done to alleviate the pain.

To remedy feelings of helplessness and hopelessness, it is advantageous if you and your chiropractor can partner in your care and treatment plan. Being an active team player in the decisions made to return your quality of life is fundamental to your well-being. Teaming up with your chiropractor gives you back a sense of control over your life and allows you to do the things you choose to do. Depression lifts, and a more positive attitude is achieved. When you take an active, participatory role in your own wellness, you begin to realize that your choices about your health matter.

Because some foods feed inflammation in the body and in turn cause pain in the neck, part of your responsibility for your health is to choose foods that help you get well. Given this knowledge, nutrition and dietary counseling will also be important for your pain relief. Dr. Wu stresses the importance of a two-way approach that includes realignment along with improvements in nutrition and dietary cleansing. He describes the importance of nutrition and cleansing through diet in this way:

> I talk with my patients about having a car that usually needs an oil filter change every three months. Well, our bodies go through so much over the years that it makes sense to put good gasoline in but also to cleanse the filters. I know that if waste is not being eliminated satisfactorily and things are not clean inside that symptoms will manifest on the outside. So by using a two-way approach, people have quicker pain relief. Even those people who have age-related high blood pressure can get off their high blood pressure medication sooner.

Conclusion

Chiropractic has been available throughout North America for at least a century. This makes it easy to find a chiropractor in nearly every city or town. However, different schools of chiropractic offer slightly different philosophies concerning treatment approaches. Some chiropractors are purists, believing that the body can heal itself with the assistance of chiropractic care alone. Others are more integrated into a complex of additional medical services offered. It is important that you work with a chiropractor who shares your views and is right for you.

More physicians are beginning to refer their clients to chiropractors, so this may be a good place to start with your decision. Otherwise, reference by word of mouth or by interview with a prospective chiropractor will be helpful. Throughout this book we will be encouraging you to check the credentials of any health-care professional you choose because choosing the right therapist is more important than hiring an electrician or plumber. Your health and well-being are at stake.

All chiropractors offer hands-on treatment of the spine, nervous system, pelvis, and joints. However, not all doctors of chiropractic can offer Dr. Wu's in-depth knowledge of nutrition. Therefore, a more detailed discussion about nutrition and the importance of healthy eating is found under the section presented by the integrative nutritional counselor.

Chapter Four: Acupuncture and Craniosacral Therapy

Maria Redinger is a massage therapist, acupuncturist, and craniosacral therapist in California.

The following quotes are from a June 18, 2012 interview with Maria. We thank Maria for her contribution to the following section on acupuncture and craniosacral therapy.

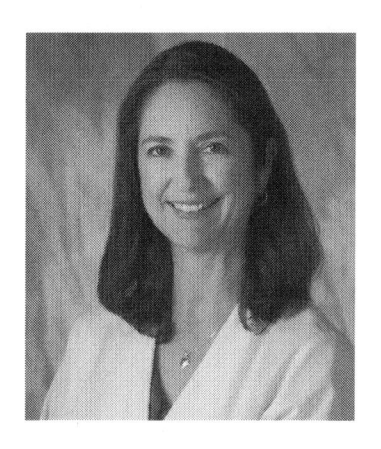

Introduction

The makings of a multitalented and caring health professional were present in Maria in childhood. At the age of five, Maria was already doing a form of massage therapy by walking on her father's back when he returned home after a long day at work.

Maria, trained as a massage therapist, acupuncturist, and craniosacral therapist, is a versatile practitioner who has been providing therapy for her clients for fifteen years. Her understanding of and compassion for her older clients is evident in her approach to their care.

What Is Acupuncture?

Acupuncture is a health-care treatment that originated in China perhaps as long as five thousand years ago. In the Chinese tradition, physicians believe that everything within and outside of our bodies affects our health: that is, the energy in our bodies, as part of nature, is constantly changing and flowing. Keeping constant change and flow in harmony both inside and outside of our bodies is the central intention of Eastern medicine.[8]

The purpose of acupuncture is to encourage the body's natural healing, improve body function, and relieve pain by unblocking congested energy pathways. The energy pathways that connect the acupuncture points are called *meridians*.

What Causes Neck Soreness from an Acupuncture View?

According to Chinese medicine, energy flows through our bodies by way of meridians or pathways. To maintain health and well-being, energy must flow freely from the inside of the body to the skin, tendons, bones, and joints. Blocked energy causes disharmony, pain, dysfunction, and disease. Maria explains neck pain from an acupuncture viewpoint when she says that,

> These meridians that run through the body are like little rivers flowing...if there's an avalanche that causes rocks and trees and debris to fall into the river that

---

[8] About.com, "Alternative Medicine" *Acupuncture,* http://www.altmedicine.about.com/cs/treatmentsad/a/acupuncture.htm (accessed 19 June 2012).

blocks the flow of the water. It's the same in the body…if somebody falls or has an accident or even isn't drinking enough water, the energy flow is impeded through the meridians and is experienced as pain. And if the blockage is there long enough, it can lead to dysfunction and disease.

The "debris" that falls into the energy channels of your body can come from many different places. One factor that may contribute to pain and loss of function is natural aging with its associated degenerative process, arthritis, including arthritic spurs that may have developed in your neck bones. Pain could be arising from the muscles that support your head and neck due to lack of movement and exercise and consequent reduction in the amount of blood circulating to your muscles and joints. Inflammation may block your energy flow, aggravate your neck muscles, and produce muscle spasms that can be very painful.

Pain can often be due to stress and worry that arises from both inside and outside of our bodies, causing tension and imbalance in the body. Therefore stress and worries can be a cause of pain and/or contribute to both the length of the pain experience and/or its severity. Poor nutrition and insufficient fluid intake can also contribute to pain or increase its felt response. All therapist address pain from a holistic perspective but acupuncturists believe that the primary source for pain is blockages of the meridians.

Differences between Men and Women

As an acupuncturist, Maria believes that women tend to experience neck pain from tension and emotional upsets far more often than men. Men tend toward physical causes such as bone and joint degeneration and dehydration due to poor fluid intake.

As we age and we have less energy to invest, it is understandable that we worry more. Family, health, and financial pressures are the major sources for anxiety, and anxiety can play a huge role in neck pain. Therefore women in particular need to have a therapist who has the time and desire to listen to their worries and provide support and encouragement. Maria understands the needs of aging adults regardless of their gender and ensures that their physical as well as emotional and spiritual needs are met. As a therapist, Maria shows her sensitivity when she says:

> The clients who come to me just want to feel better. I think that's a big part of the therapy, too. Letting clients talk, listening to what they have to say you know: whatever's on their mind, their problems. They have 100 percent attention in the time that they're with me, and that in itself is worth a lot.

The hands-on nature of holistic practice allows time to listen to clients while providing therapy. Having a listener is an invaluable experience for older adults, especially when they are living with pain.

What You Can Expect When You Visit an Acupuncturist

As a holistic practitioner, an acupuncturist is interested in the energy flow through your whole body. Obviously, she will ask you for your health history, including past and present illness as well as a description of your current pain experience. In acupuncture, each person is an individual and is treated accordingly.

Because stress plays such a large role in neck pain, your acupuncturist will also be interested in your environment, the quality of your work life (if applicable), and your home life. She will ask about your current lifestyle, such as your use of prescribed and over-the-counter medications and eating and exercise habits.

Your descriptions form the basis for her understanding of where your energy is blocked so that she will know at which points along your body's meridians to place acupuncture needles. Once a diagnosis is made, very fine needles will be inserted at predetermined points along your meridian channels in order to unblock your obstructed energy, allowing it to flow freely and your pain to be diminished. For example, pain in your shoulders almost always comes from your neck. Your acupuncturist would insert a needle, or needles, along the meridian points that move energy between your neck and shoulders.

The number of acupuncture treatments you receive will be based on your unique requirements. The decision to end or continue treatment is always made in collaboration between you and your acupuncturist.

Partnering with Your Acupuncturist

Your therapist is interested in what you feel both during a treatment and between treatments. This kind of information will help her understand where blockages still exist or if new concerns have arisen that need to be addressed.

If you are someone who eats a very healthy diet and exercises regularly, your needs will be very different from those of someone who has had many health challenges and is not as physically fit. Your well-being determines your readiness for treatment and the length and number of treatments that will be right for you.

For example, physically fit adults who follow their practitioner's advice will respond more quickly to acupuncture treatments and thus need fewer visits. More energetic, they are more likely to follow advice that may include simply increasing water intake, reducing the amount of coffee they drink, or choosing from a variety of different foods to add to their diet.

If you are in a more frail condition, you will more likely require a longer program of treatment and more acupuncturist visits. In such a case, you can effectively partner with your acupuncturist by engaging in a moderate exercise program, eating a more balanced diet, and drinking plenty of water. Again, your acupuncturist will suggest changes that benefit you now and in the future. The key is to stay with the process of treatment by keeping an open mind and trying new approaches such as the following suggested by Maria:

> Very gentle, slow movements that help to keep energy channels open... that can make a big difference in overall health...tai chi...or even some light yoga....There are some individuals teaching yoga for seniors now. Depending on their ability, seniors can even do yoga exercises from a chair or wheelchair for those who are wheelchair bound...any kind of movement exercise... breathing...even just breathing will help a lot, too.

For those of you who are frail, any additions to your daily routine will take vitality, and you may be feeling that yours is very low. Your acupuncturist will be aware of your energy levels and will take a gentle, encouraging approach. Also be gentle with yourself and recognize that relieving your neck pain may take just a little longer than it does for someone who is more physically hearty.

Remember that you and your therapist are partners in the relief of your pain and in your return to the activities that you most enjoy. You will heal faster and more completely when you recognize that you need each other along your journey to pain relief. You are partners, each relying on the other to do his or her best job. Most importantly, you need to trust and respect each other, something that takes time. Maria highlights how she builds relationships with her clients:

> I have a very gentle touch, and that seems to attract seniors to me, and I love working with them as well. I love hearing their stories. I get a lot out of it. It's a two-way street. They get a lot from me working on them, and I get a lot from them. I love listening to their stories and their lives, the things that they've done in their lives; I just love it.

Living with pain can make us fearful of being touched, especially on the affected area. Having your pain experience valued in such a way as to inspire gentleness in how your therapist touches your body and your heart adds an invaluable dimension to partnership. It is an added bonus when we realize how much our therapist is dedicated to our healing.

What Is Craniosacral Therapy?

A hands-on, gentle treatment, craniosacral therapy (CST) is an approach that releases tension to reduce pain and immobility and improve total body health. CST positively impacts the way your body functions as well as your emotional health.

What Causes Neck Soreness from a CST Viewpoint?

Chronic neck pain adds to our experience of daily stress, strain, and tension, which causes muscles to tighten and contract and, in turn, increase pain. As Maria explains, we often underestimate the effect that tension can have:

> Tension in the neck is not confined to the neck…it goes right up into the cranium and inside the meninges that cover the brain. They also tighten up. That can affect mental processing and the circulation of cerebral spinal fluid (the fluid that surrounds, protects, and nourishes the brain and spinal cord).

Stop for a moment and check the amount of tension that you carry in your muscles. Are your teeth clenched? Are your shoulders raised?

When muscles tighten, the stress places additional strain on your body's connective tissue. The function of connective tissue is to support and connect your body's various parts and organs. Pressure on your central nervous system and spine is also increased, causing pain and restricting activity. Holding tension in our muscles can, over time, develop into a pain pattern because muscles have memory.

Maria notes, "Patterns of strain or tension are held in the connective tissue that covers every muscle, every organ, and every body cavity from head to toe. Therefore, tension reduction results in improved circulation, blood and cerebral spinal fluid flows. Clients feel better, and think more clearly."

What You Can Expect When You Visit a CST Practitioner

Your craniosacral therapist will want to know what has brought you to her for help. She may not require as complete a history as other therapists, but she will need background information concerning your condition. In a typical craniosacral session, you will be asked to lie down on a massage table. The practitioner will place his or her hands gently and lightly on your body and tune into your body's unique rhythm. The same light, soothing touch is used in various places on your body to release any tension felt throughout your connective tissue.

The first thing that you may notice is a sense of deep relaxation that lasts throughout the session and even longer. As your tension is released, you will begin to feel more centered in contrast to a previous feeling of pain-related anxiety or irritability. You will also feel a decrease in the amount and quality of pain that you were experiencing on arrival. Gentle though it is, the release of tension is intensely healing.

Partnering with Your CST Practitioner

Partnering with your CST practitioner means that you each have a job to do. Your therapist provides therapy specific to your presenting condition and educates and instructs you on how to receive the most benefit from her therapy. Your job is to follow her instructions.

Taking responsibility for your job in a partnership boosts your self-esteem and increases your confidence that your pain can and will be alleviated. The first task that is asked of you is to drink plenty of water because older adults can easily become dehydrated. If you are someone who only drinks water when you take medications, you can make a huge difference simply by drinking additional water or other fluids throughout the day. Coffee is not recommended because it can dehydrate the body and add to your problem.

If you happen to be one of those people who do not like the taste of water, you can try filtered water or bottled water. Some water-bottling companies make home deliveries, or you can buy bottled water at the grocery store. Adding a slice of lemon to a glass of water not only improves its taste, but it can also aid digestion.

Exercise is of utmost importance to increase blood flow and oxygen delivery to your muscles. Slow, gentle movements count as exercise. Your CST therapist may encourage you to walk more, perform gentle stretching when arising from a seated or a lying position, or join a senior's yoga or tai chi group. All movement counts because exercise improves mood and decreases stress.

Because no major lifestyle change is easy, you may feel the need to discuss your worries and concerns over with your craniosacral therapist, a family member, your spiritual advisor, or anyone who is willing to listen and help you find your answers.

Although craniosacral work is deeply calming, re-entering places of stress after treatment will interfere with the healing properties of therapy. You, too, must be aware of yourself as a multifaceted human being and be willing to address all areas of your life. When you are open to working on the emotional, spiritual, and cognitive aspects of your neck-pain experience, you can partner with your holistic practitioner more effectively.

Conclusion

Acupuncture and craniosacral therapy work in two different ways to relieve neck pain. While acupuncture uses very thin needles to unblock obstructed energy flows, craniosacral therapy is more hands-on, influences your connective tissue, and is more relaxing as the therapy is being carried out. Finding a therapist with expertise in both areas is an exceptional experience.

If there is no craniosacral therapist in your area, you might find other practices that release stress, such as breathing exercises, yoga, and qigong, helpful. Everyone should give consideration to counseling because having a listener is very helpful for addressing the underlying source of worries and concerns.

ALICE KASSEL'S STORY

This section was volunteered by Alice Kassel who offered to share her story to encourage others, who are living with neck pain. As Ms. Kassel's therapist, Maria Redinger partnered with Ms. Kassel to gain mastery over her pain. Ms. Kassel's hope is that her story will serve as inspiration to others who are currently suffering with neck pain. Her story, as written by Maria Redinger, is gratefully accepted as an exemplar of the power of partnership and as Ms. Kassel's openness to trying holistic therapies for relief of her neck pain.

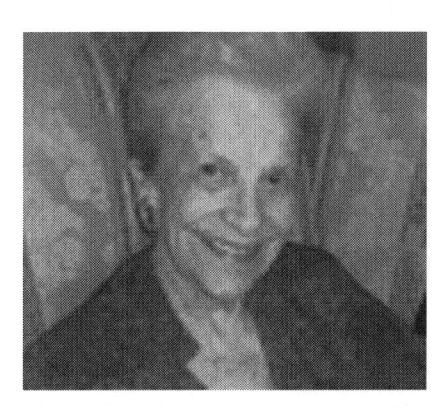

Alice is ninety-three years old. She is a resident of Bridgecreek Retirement Center in West Covina, California. I first met her about five years ago. A friend of mine was teaching yoga at Bridgecreek, and one of her students, Ms. Kassel, was experiencing neck pain. My friend thought I could help her with massage.

I met Alice at her home and we began our work together. As I gently massaged her neck and shoulders, I could feel the tightness on the right side of her neck and shoulders. Alice described the area as "very painful." Even more disconcerting to her was the fact that her medical doctor's examination showed no evidence of an underlying disease process. As I began to better understand

Alice, we began to talk about situations that could be causing her distress. As we chatted, she mentioned that she had a gentleman friend whom she was very fond of, but he caused her great distress whenever he acted in a certain way. Together, we realized that the source of her neck and shoulder pain was rooted in the nature of her relationship. Alice and I knew her pain was very real, even though her physician was unable to find a disease-related cause.

We chatted the entire time I massaged her, and by the end of the session, Alice had a big smile on her face—and no more neck pain. She said that she would talk to the residents and get them interested in massage also. Well, talk she did. I have been going to Bridgecreek every month since then to provide massage, and now acupuncture as well, at a rate the residents can afford.

Over the years that I have known Alice, she has had several bouts of neck pain, always in the same area and always associated with stress due to relationships. With the most recent occurrence, Alice's neck pain was on the right side, and she rated it an eight out of ten, with ten being an extreme degree of pain. The discomfort was constant, and the severity of pain would increase and decrease from day to day. Alice described it as "an aching, continual pain." Her doctor gave her medicinal patches, which she said helped for the first four days, but then stopped working. Alice noticed that the pain was worse when she spoke to a particular gentleman friend. She said, "For a while I felt fine. But the minute I would get stressful thoughts, I'd feel pain."

Alice found that prayer helped her to get rid of the problem. She told me, "Believe in your prayer." Alice shared, "Massage and prayer is the best thing of all. No pills have helped me. It started a long time ago. Stress brings it on…men…relatives. When I say "no more men!" then "I'm OK." Alice then added, "When I gave up trying to get a certain person to like me, I felt better." She also offered, "It helps to talk about it."

Chapter Five: Natural Medicine

Dr. Linda Henderson is a doctor of natural medicine and homeopathy and owner and head practitioner of Halton Holistic Healthcare in Ontario, Canada. She is also a Reiki master with an advanced degree in traditional Chinese medicine and acupuncture, a diploma in naturopathy, and numerous certificates in hypnotherapy, therapeutic touch, kinesiology, healing touch, aromatherapy, and reflexology.

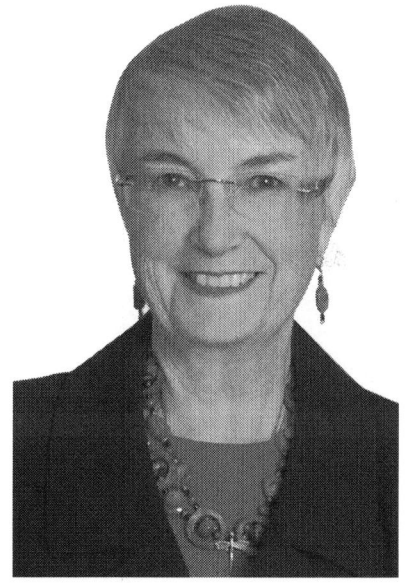

Dr. Henderson is also the director of training and educational development and a senior instructor for the College of International Holistic Studies.

The following quotes were provided by Dr. Henderson on May 28, 2012. We thank Dr. Henderson for her contribution to this section on doctors of natural medicine.

Introduction

Dr. Henderson was just a teenager when her teaching skills were recognized and valued by the Windsor School Board. Sponsored by the board, she graduated from the Windsor Teachers' College in Ontario and began teaching at age eighteen. Her love of teaching has continuously informed her career in health care so that one could best describe Linda as an extraordinary teacher-healer.

The healing part of her practice was inspired by her medical doctor, who played a major role in helping Linda to succeed. She describes him as having the biggest heart of anyone she has ever worked with in the medical profession. What he modeled for Linda was that the practice of medicine is simultaneously an art and a science and that one cannot be abandoned in favor of the other. Most importantly, Linda is a lifelong learner who has a sharp and curious mind and, through her perpetual pursuit of knowledge, a sincere commitment to helping her clients heal.

What Is a Doctor of Natural Medicine?

Doctors of natural medicine are multifaceted health-care professionals trained in basic medical sciences as well as complementary medicine. They use their extensive education and training to treat the total person—body, mind, and spirit. Their practice covers many treatment modalities that are based in nature and are all-encompassing. Doctors of natural medicine do not prescribe drugs; rather, they use remedies such as yoga, breathing exercises, and meditation in conjunction with herbs and tinctures from traditional Chinese medicine, homeopathy, and botanical medicine to relieve a client's symptoms and restore him to health and well-being.

Practitioners of homeopathic medicine believe that "like cures like"—that an illness can be deregulated by a substance that produces symptoms similar to those of the illness in healthy people.

Homeopaths also accept the notion of minimal dose, that the lower the dose of a prescribed mixture, the greater its effectiveness. Like those of traditional Chinese medicine, homeopathic remedies come from natural plants and herbs but may also include other nutrients from nature such as crushed bees.[9]

As you will note from Linda's credentials, doctors of natural medicine are highly educated and not limited in their scope of practice. Doctors of natural medicine must meet standards of practice established by the World Organization of Natural Medicine Practitioners (WONMP).

What Causes Neck Soreness from a Doctor of Natural Medicine View?

Because of their wide scope of practice, doctors of natural medicine consider multiple factors for the underlying causes of neck soreness. Linda provided us with several examples of underlying causes for neck pain.

When considering how human beings work, walk, and sleep, we become aware of how much posture plays a role in neck pain. Although workplaces are designed today as ergonomically appropriate environments, when older adults were employed, this was not the case. Sitting hunched over a typewriter, computer, or sewing machine all day, filing, taking notes, or engaging in other activities that require keeping one's head down all greatly contribute to current neck pain in older adults. Police officers and taxi drivers, who spend long hours sitting in car seats poorly designed for human spines, can have serious neck problems later in life. Wear, tear, and tension on workers' shoulders and spines will also challenge their spines and necks later in life. Consider the heavy and repetitive activities involved in construction work.

---

[9] National Center for Complementary and Alternative Medicine, "Health Info," *Homeopathy: An Introduction*, http://www.nccam.nih.gov/health/homeopathy (accessed 29 May 2012).

Add to these factors accidents, falls, and motor vehicle mishaps and you can begin to see how complex the causes of neck pain can be.

The way we walk, bend, lift, carry, and sleep has implications for spinal health. People who lack confidence are inclined to walk with their heads down or their backs hunched. Over time, these postures will cause structural changes and pain. People who walk in a way that is unbalanced and those who sleep on their side without a pillow between their knees are also liable to have neck problems in later life because posture can, over time, change the position of vertebrae.

Eating an acidic diet or a diet high in carbohydrates can contribute to neck pain, as can dental practices involving the use of mercury to repair teeth. Dr. Henderson explains, "Every tooth in our body is connected to a vertebra and to a muscle and an organ… everything is interconnected, so the source of pain may not be just one thing. Take a look at where those mercury fillings are. Which came first, the mercury fillings or the neck pain?" Dr. Henderson's words remind us that we need to be aware of what we are putting into our mouths.

As other holistic practitioners have informed us, stress is a major contributing factor to neck pain. Dr. Henderson agrees:

> When stressed we tend to raise our shoulders up around our ears, which actually tightens all the muscles in the neck region. Once they start to tighten and pull, that will often throw the spinal vertebrae out of alignment, and then you're left with a sore neck.

In addition, Linda speaks to the difficulty and consequent stress that many older people have giving voice to their needs. If we fear speaking up even on our own behalf, our worries cannot be heard and our needs cannot be addressed. Feeling fully heard is the forerunner of trust, and trust is the basis for all caring relationships.

Differences between Men and Women

Dr. Henderson has found in her practice that, older females, reluctant to burden others, are less likely than males to share their pain experiences. This, Dr. Henderson explains, causes women to "become chronic before they actually need to." When we delay seeking attention for pain, we risk doing permanent damage to our joints and tissues, which means that the underlying problem has become chronic.

The propensity of women to be primary caregivers even into old age can put them at risk for neck problems. If caregiving is stressful for young women, it is even more so for aging women. Having lived a lifetime of putting others first, women may need to share and build feelings of self-worth with a counselor or spiritual advisor in order to break old patterns of giving without being able to receive. Anyone with neck pain deserves the time and attention necessary to help her find comfort and healing.

Other challenges for aging women are symptoms associated with menopause, such as lowered libido, hot flashes, and their greater leaning toward arthritis. When the myriad of contributing factors for neck pain in older adults is considered, one can appreciate the knowledge and skills that a doctor of natural medicine brings to the health-care partnership.

What You Can Expect When You Visit a Doctor of Natural Medicine

Because neck pain is your presenting symptom, when you arrive at the office of a doctor of natural medicine, the first treatment you will receive is one that will relieve your pain. Only when your pain is relieved will you have the vitality to commit to the lifestyle changes necessary to keep your pain manageable.

There are a number of pain-relieving treatments and several lifestyle changes that a doctor of natural medicine may offer you, depending on her assessment of your overall health. Expect the assessment to be detailed and comprehensive, covering your physical, emotional, cognitive, and spiritual well-being. Once the doctor of natural medicine has formed her diagnosis, she will present therapies and lifestyle changes unique to your individual needs and expectations.

Dr. Henderson uses a specialized machine called an electro-interstitial scan (E.I.S) for diagnostic purposes, and your doctor of natural medicine may do the same. Use of the machine is noninvasive, pain-free, and provides vast amounts of information about you that is invaluable for diagnostic purposes. Such information includes physiological data that provide the doctor with information about your hormone and mineral levels, blood gasses, brain neurotransmitters and more.

Once your pain is more bearable, you and your doctor will begin the work of changing old habits in the way that you eat, exercise, and relax. It is a good idea to bring your spouse or other family member with you to consult with your doctor because changing a lifestyle pattern will affect everyone you live with. For example, a man who is having neck pain may be given a specific diet, but it is his wife who prepares his meals. If she has been present during her husband's assessment and has been included in the plan, she will more likely support the changes when shopping and cooking. A change in one person creates a ripple effect throughout one's family and extended family. You will need the support of your family and friends as you embark on your journey back to health.

Partnering with Your Doctor of Natural Medicine

Like all holistic healers, a doctor of natural medicine will conduct a comprehensive examination of the total you. Here, then, is the opportunity to use your voice and be fully heard. The treatment plan that your doctor develops for you is only as good as the information that you provide. As a partner in your recovery from pain, your doctor should be aware of everything and anything about you that will aid in a diagnosis of your condition and an understanding of the root cause for your pain. Remember that each client the doctor sees is a unique and special individual and, as such, is highly regarded.

Because your doctor will be looking for underlying causes for your neck pain, she may prescribe remedies such as a more alkaline diet, glucosamine, and minerals. As has often been stated, one of the best ways that you can help is by drinking more water. Dr. Henderson notes that, "the older generation are not big water-drinkers."

Neck stretches, yoga, and shoulder rolls are all exercises that release tension and neck strain and help strengthen and soften your neck muscles. Your doctor of natural medicine may teach you these exercises or refer you to a physiotherapist or yoga/pilates/qigong instructor. She may also send you to other health professionals, like a chiropractor, if she believes that a spinal adjustment is indicated. It is vital that you follow your doctor's directions and comply with her treatment plan.

Finally, through the practice of yoga and meditation, you can contribute much to your recovery because these practices relieve stress and tension as well as help you to remain calm in the face of life's stressors, whether associated with your relationships, finances, or health. By accepting your role as partner in your journey to well-being, you make the work of your doctor of natural medicine much easier and your return to health much quicker.

Conclusion

Doctors of natural medicine are educated and trained in a number of health disciplines; therefore, they have many different tools to help you overcome your neck pain. However, if you choose to engage a doctor of natural medicine as a partner in wellness, you must be prepared to make the lifestyle changes recommended to you. An open mind and a willingness to take charge of your life will greatly enhance your success.

Chapter Six: Reflexology and Bowen Therapy

Jack Marriott has been a certified reflexologist since the early 1990s and was also among the first Canadians trained in ear reflexology. Co-owner, co-principal, and registrar of the Universal College of Reflexology, Jack is also recognized as an internationally known speaker and seminar leader. He is involved in continuing professional development, and through the college, provides programs consistent with the requirements of the reflexology accreditation boards in North America.

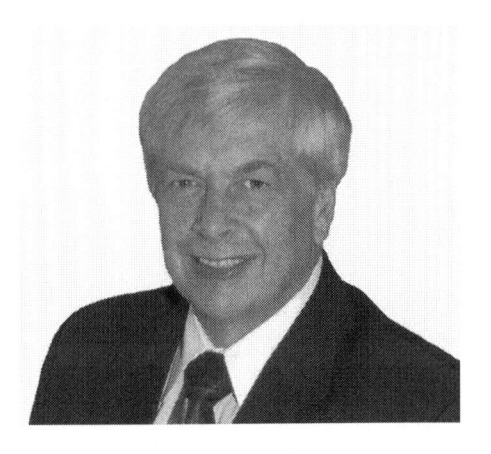

Jack continues to practice, teach, and write in Parksville on Vancouver Island, British Columbia, Canada.

The following quotes were provided by Jack on July 27, 2012. We thank Jack Marriott for his contribution to the following section on reflexology and Bowen therapy.

Introduction

Jack had a very interesting journey on his way to becoming a reflexologist and Bowen therapist. He was on a physical and spiritual path—physical because of his love of sports and spiritual because throughout his life he has used what he has learned to enrich the lives of others.

All athletes are subject to injury, often serious. In Jack's case, some of his injuries led to hospitalization and surgery. Subsequent recovery from his more serious injuries is described by Jack as "very stressful." He worried about his capacity to continue sports and encountered numerous side effects from the surgery itself as well as from prescribed medications. Needless to say, after a number of hospitalizations, he had a much better understanding of his own body and what he needed to do to return to health and well-being.

Like many dedicated athletes, in the decade between his thirties and forties, Jack began to experience injury-related pain and discomfort. To complicate matters, he also developed a whole-body health challenge that resulted in pain and swelling in his hands, fingers, and joints. At the same time that Jack was suffering from his own health challenge, his mother became ill, an illness that would take Jack further along his spiritual path.

> In the days before she passed, I just got this intuitive, insightful, inspirational sense from my mom...that I have to do something different with my life but I wasn't sure what that was. So I had this inspiration from my Mom, and it led me to question, "What can I do that has something to do with drugless therapy, alternative practice, and things like that?" ...I had never had an

alternative medicine session before. Nothing. I just had this sort of belief that it was right. So that's what I did, and that started my career in reflexology.

Fingers and thumbs are the tools of reflexology, and despite the pain in his hands and fingers, Jack persisted in making a career of his newly found vocation. Jack's success orientation learned from sports and his newfound reflexology knowledge became the vehicles that ultimately healed him of his own health challenge. He describes his healing process:

> Here's the interesting thing: within a year or two, all of a sudden I realized that I wasn't in pain anymore. My knuckles looked normal; I could touch them with no problem. I could even wear a ring. I thought, Wow, this is amazing! And it wasn't because I was receiving reflexology—I wasn't. It was because I was *giving* reflexology. Now isn't that interesting? I was actually giving myself a reflexology session every time I worked on somebody else.

What Is Reflexology?

The practice of reflexology is as old as ancient Egypt. Tomb reliefs found in pyramids dating to the sixth dynasty (ca. 2450 BC) show two men seated and receiving treatments on their hands and feet.[10]

A complementary health-care practice, reflexology involves the application of pressure to "zones," or reflexes found on specific areas on the body. These reflex areas are reflected on the feet, hands, and ears. When pressure is applied to these zones, a physical change is initiated in the corresponding regions of the body—glands, organs, all body structures. These physiological changes stimulate the body's natural electrical energy system to clear any

---

10 "Egyptian Footwork: Therapy, Beauty, Foot Rub or All Three?" http://www.foot-reflexologist.com/EGYPT_1.HTM (accessed 6 Jan. 2013).

blockages within corresponding body regions. The notion of clearing blockages closely resembles the release of blockages in acupuncture.

As a holistic therapy, the process of reflexology works on the entire body, alleviating stress as it returns the body to its natural balance (homeostasis), consequently improving blood circulation and oxygenation. Jack explains this holistic practice:

> There may be a combination of things happening in the body, and because the neck is the weakest link, that's where the pain is happening. Without concentrating just on the neck reflexes, we address everything that is happening in the body. Reflexology works from the inside out and is probably one of the only therapies, with the exception of acupuncture, that does that. Every other therapy works from the outside in, so this is a real key to reflexology being a wonderful type of therapy.

Reflexology is considered to be a complementary therapy inasmuch as it is holistic in nature and can be used in conjunction with other therapies including conventional medicine, physiotherapy, counseling, and the use of drug therapy, and as a postsurgical healing strategy. Jack informs us that complementary medicine is moving toward a more integrated approach with other therapies, including allopathic medicine. That is, health-care providers are coming together in collaborative practice. This is an important move as working collaboratively informs a true partnership among health-care professionals and can only benefit you, our client and partner.

What Causes Neck Soreness from a Reflexology and Bowen Therapy View?

Reflexology and Bowen therapy agree on the causal bases for neck pain: age, injury, poor posture, dehydration, pollution, stress, diet, and exercise. The following provides information on each of these underlying causes.

Injuries due to falls, accidents, sports, or motor vehicle mishaps and age-related conditions such as osteoporosis, osteoarthritis, and spinal stenosis all contribute to the progression of neck problems and pain in older adults.

We live and work very differently from the way our ancestors did. Our lifestyles tend to be much more sedentary. We sit for long periods of time in front of the computer or television. We travel long distances in our cars, sit in traffic, and worry that we'll be late in reaching our destination. Sitting for long periods puts pressure on the spine, neck and shoulders. Worry tightens back muscles and only adds to the strain.

Some of us notice that we are walking with hunched backs or rounded shoulders. Reflexologists believe that poor posture over the long term is one of the main contributors to neck pain. Sitting for extended periods as well as a lifetime of poor overall posture is responsible for our experience of pain in later years. Our bodies need to move and exercise at all ages.

Factors such as the accumulation of toxins in our muscles from dehydration, poor eating habits, and environmental pollutants are at the root of neck pain. In particular, lack of sufficient fluid intake directly affects the neck and spine. Jack explains, "Nearly all people don't drink enough water. The jelly in the vertebrae that keeps it together is almost all water, so we've found that a lot of people with chronic back pain and chronic neck pain are really dehydrated no matter what age."

The jellylike substance in the center of the vertebral discs that Jack refers to acts like a water sac or pillow to distribute pressure and absorb shock within each vertebral disc. The intervertebral discs, together, allow for range of motion through the spinal column. Because water makes up most of the gelatinous core, you can appreciate the importance of drinking plenty of water.

Eating poorly can mean that insufficient nourishment is being provided to maintain important structures in your muscles, spine, and neck bones. Nutrition is of major importance as we age.

Increasing water intake and eating a healthier organic diet can also help eliminate environmental toxins. To assist in your understanding about the importance of nutrition, make sure you read the section provided by Paul Martin Jr., integrative nutritionist and health counselor.

Differences between Men and Women

As we age, some of us tend to lose calcium and trace minerals from our bones, causing a subsequent breakdown in bone density. When bone loss is just beginning, the condition is known as osteopenia, but when the loss is advanced, it is called osteoporosis. While osteoporosis can occur in men, it is more prominent in women; for either gender, it is very serious. Appropriate exercise, especially the use of weights, can make a dramatic difference for both genders, especially when combined with a nutritional diet and increased water intake.

Women, who are more accustomed to grocery shopping and preparing meals, may find it easier to eat a balanced diet to stave off early bone loss. Loss of estrogen production in women can lead to osteoporosis, thus the importance of a yearly medical checkup and bone density examination as ordered by your physician. However, men, especially single men or widowers living alone, may find this more difficult.

What You Can Expect When You Visit a Reflexologist

To understand your individual health challenge, the reflexologist will ask many questions about your health history including when your pain began, what exacerbates your pain, what medications you may be taking, if you have been to another health professional for treatment, and what measures you have taken yourself to relieve your neck pain. For example, the reflexologist will be interested in whether applying heat to your neck helps or whether certain activities increase your pain. All of this information is useful because reflexology complements other therapies and interventions, such as chiropractic and drug use.

Reflexologists are careful to prepare an environment in which their clients feel comfortable and relaxed. The atmosphere is clean, quiet, and conducive to your comfort. Usually, you will be asked to sit in a recliner because it is most comfortable, but reflexology can be administered to clients who are sitting up or lying down. Your comfort is of utmost importance, so you can choose whether your time with the reflexologist will be quiet time, with limited talking, or if you want to converse to share concerns with your therapist.

Recall that our emotions can lead us into pain. For example, avoiding difficult relationships where self-assertion would be useful can virtually give you a pain in the neck in the absence of any injury, degenerative disease, or illness. Remember that tension and stress play a huge role in your pain experience.

Although they are not counselors, reflexologists tend to be very good listeners, so you should use this time to get your needs met; this includes talking over any concerns and asking any questions you may have. The treatment, on both feet, will usually last roughly forty minutes to an hour. Do not be upset if you fall asleep; many people do.

Your reflexologist will most likely work on your feet, but he may also choose to work on your hands or ears. Consequently, he will complete a thorough examination before he begins.

A firm pressure is used when working the foot reflexes, but not enough to inflict pain. The reflexologist will check with you periodically to see if you are experiencing discomfort. Perhaps he will use a scale from one to ten (one being acceptable and ten being past your pain threshold) to gauge your comfort level with his use of pressure. Note that reflexology is not a foot massage. Your body's natural healing process needs to be stimulated by a certain amount of pressure during reflexology. The pressure stimulates your body's healing response.

Partnering with Your Reflexologist

Seeking help from any holistic practitioner requires a willingness to work in partnership because taking a holistic approach involves working the entire body, not simply your neck. As a partner in your return to well-being, you can do several things, starting with increasing your intake of water and committing to well-balanced and nutritional eating.

In addition, try to avoid sitting for long periods of time. If you have a hobby (reading, watching TV, or doing needlework, or jigsaw puzzles) that requires long periods of sitting, set the alarm on the stove for thirty minutes, and when it sounds, get up, walk around, and reset the alarm. This practice will ensure that you give yourself breaks in which you bring your head back to a more normal position. In addition, doing gentle neck stretches before returning to your activity can be most helpful. If you are also seeing a physiotherapist, she can show you which exercises would be useful. More importantly, you should commit to exercising—walking, cycling, yoga, qigong—for at least thirty minutes a day. Our bodies need to move kinetically every day. So get out there and move.

You should arrive at each appointment with clean feet and well-trimmed toenails. Be sure to discuss any foot problems such as arthritic spurs, fasciitis, blisters, and so on with your reflexologist. Make sure to inform your reflexologist if you have any allergies to perfumes so that he can select a lotion, oil, or cream that will not compromise your visit. During treatment, inform him, using the scale of one to ten, about your pain threshold so that he can adjust his pressure accordingly.

Between visits, continuing your therapy with your physical therapist, medical doctor, counselor, spiritual advisor, or other health-care provider can only help you to progress more quickly. Always remember that you and your reflexologist are partners, each with a responsibility to the other to do your best so that he can attend to you and you can heal.

When you have lived with pain for a long time, you may be wary of therapies that directly touch or manipulate the painful area. Fear of further pain is an emotional and totally understandable response to treatment. You simply may be unwilling to accept any more pain. But fear can block the effectiveness of treatment and leave you believing that nothing works. The good news is that reflexology treatments involve the feet, as far away from your neck as possible. For many, this alone provides relief and encourages follow-through on their treatment plan.

What Is Bowen Therapy?

Bowen therapy involves a series of gentle movements to mobilize the soft tissue component of connective tissue, which covers every organ, muscle, and body cavity, called the fascia. The Bowen therapist works with the client by using a series of very specific movements aimed at restoring the self-healing mechanism of the body. Each movement may take from ten seconds to a minute. This technique involves using the fingers and thumbs to gently move the muscles and tissues. Bowen therapy impacts the musculoskeletal system, the viscera, and the nerves and can work very well for conditions causing pain and discomfort including back, neck, hip, and shoulder pain.[11]

What You Can Expect When You Visit a Bowen Therapist

There are two principles that apply explicitly to Bowen therapy. The first principle states that less is more, which serves to allow the client's body and brain to absorb the work of the Bowen therapist.

---

11 Medical Dictionary, "Bowen Technique," *Methodology*, http://www.medical-dictionary.thefreedictionary.com (accessed 3 Aug. 2012).

> So with Bowen therapy, we do a series of moves that are very specific...And when we are finished, we then leave the room where the client is and come back no sooner than two minutes, and then we do the next series of moves and leave again. The reason [for leaving] is that the body must absorb what we've done, so we give the body time to do that. Once the session begins, you do not promote conversation; you want to minimize interference with the client.

The pauses between movement sets and the gentleness of the treatment are what make Bowen therapy unique. In this process, the body has time and opportunity to use its intelligence for restoration and stabilization.

Just as the therapist does not interfere with the client, the client also does nothing to interfere with the energetic changes in her body as a result of the session. Bowen therapy continues to work for several days after treatment. Therefore, the client is asked to avoid any activities that might require energy expenditure. For example, you are advised to avoid any additional therapies such as Reiki or chiropractic and to decline sports, strenuous exercise, and—given that there is a lot of energy in hot water—even a hot shower. Engaging in any such activities can overload the brain with too much information and may undo any of the progress gained from the first session. The notion of protecting the brain from too much information at once and allowing it time to respond confirms the second principle of Bowen therapy, healing occurs from the head downward. This means that healing begins with and in the brain, both physically and emotionally.

Before commencing the session, the Bowen therapist will observe the gait and alignment of the client and check a series of ranges of motion. Following the session, he will repeat this assessment. Although Bowen therapy is a gentle, noninvasive therapy, it requires the therapist to move up the spine and into the neck area. With seniors, the position may be taxing, but good results can be produced by having older adults sit upright. Serious age-related bone conditions such as osteoporosis may contraindicate Bowen therapy for an older adult. Your Bowen therapist can best assess your candidacy for treatment.

One week following the Bowen therapy session, the client is asked to return for the second session even if she believes that the first treatment solved all of her problems. The first treatment tends to balance the body in order to begin the healing process. At least one subsequent treatment is necessary to complete healing; however, chronic conditions may require several treatments. There is no negotiation concerning the second session because at least two sessions are required for treatment to be effective.

Partnering with Your Bowen Therapist

The three most important actions that you can take to work effectively with your Bowen therapist are to (1) keep hydrated by drinking plenty of water every day, (2) comply with the requirement to return in one week after your initial treatment, and (3) follow through on the direction to avoid additional energy-draining activities between visits.

Just as you would with a reflexologist, share your health and pain history, pain threshold, and any other information that will help your therapist to work with you. Again, you and your Bowen practitioner are in a partnership whose purpose is to move the total you back to health and well-being.

Conclusion

While reflexology, as a complementary health practice, works with other therapies such as physiotherapy, allopathic medicine, and natural medicine, Bowen therapy as alternative practice stands alone with the exception of continuing prescribed medications.

Each therapy has different requirements, but both have much to offer older adults in terms of pain relief. Your willingness to consider different approaches from various practitioners to relieve your neck pain or discomfort is vital. Any decision to consult with a holistic practitioner requires a readiness from you to engage in a wellness partnership. In this regard, an informed decision advantages you, the client and partner.

Chapter Seven: Yoga

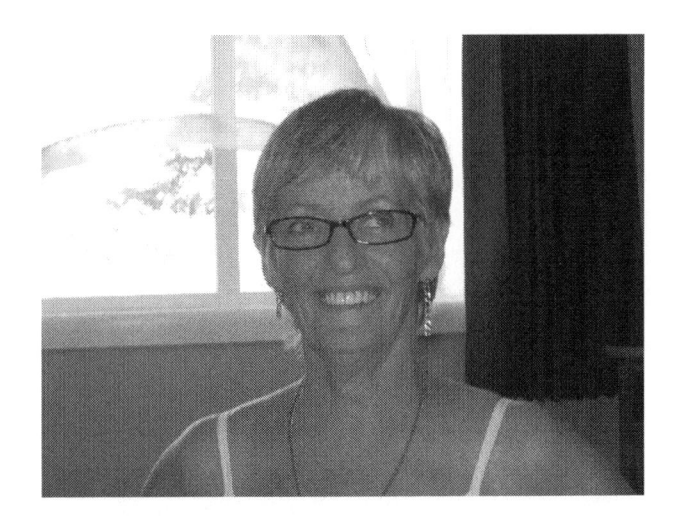

*A*dele Tedesco is a wonderful, vibrant woman who owns her own in-home mobile computer service and repair business. She has a passion for life and a way of lightening hearts and touching souls. We thank Ms. Tedesco for her contribution to the following section on yoga and for her dedication to helping others who also suffer with neck pain.

Adele Tedesco's Story

In my early thirties, I woke up one morning with a very stiff neck. It kept getting worse until I finally decided to go to the doctor. He did an examination and sent me for X-rays. The results were inconclusive, so he just told me to take Tylenol and rest it.

Eventually it got so bad that my right arm was curled up to my chest and I couldn't raise my chin. Out of desperation, I went to a chiropractor. This relieved the stiffness, and I was able to move my neck and shoulder gingerly. I just became very cautious after that with my neck. But as you would guess, the pain returned again and again. For years I suffered with this. I was going to the chiropractor regularly, and I would receive some relief, but it never did much to correct the problem and keep it away.

As the years advanced, I became despondent about this weakness of mine, and it greatly interfered in my life. In my fifties the chiropractor took X-rays, and this time I was told I had arthritis in several of my cervical vertebrae. I started going to a physiotherapist, and, in addition to the treatments she gave me, I was encouraged to do several exercises geared toward strengthening the neck and shoulder muscles. This resulted in more improvement, but it never really got rid of the problem. It just kept it at bay a little longer.

In my middle fifties I decided to do something serious about my problem, so I joined a yoga class. I practiced Iyengar yoga for six years, but I can honestly tell you that I saw an improvement within months, if not weeks. Keeping up my yoga reduced my pain level from ten to two or better. I went to yoga classes twice or three times a week, and the neck and shoulder strengthened to a point where I came to believe I had no arthritis in my neck. And we all know there is no cure for arthritis. I added massage to my regimen a few years later, and with the massage came even more improvement.

Actual proof, to me, that yoga is the answer to some health issues is the fact that I measured three-quarters of an inch taller after one year of yoga. Yoga has given me a much healthier body and an improved disposition. It has given me the ability to do what I choose physically, without pain.

Chapter Eight: Clinical Hypnotherapy and Reiki

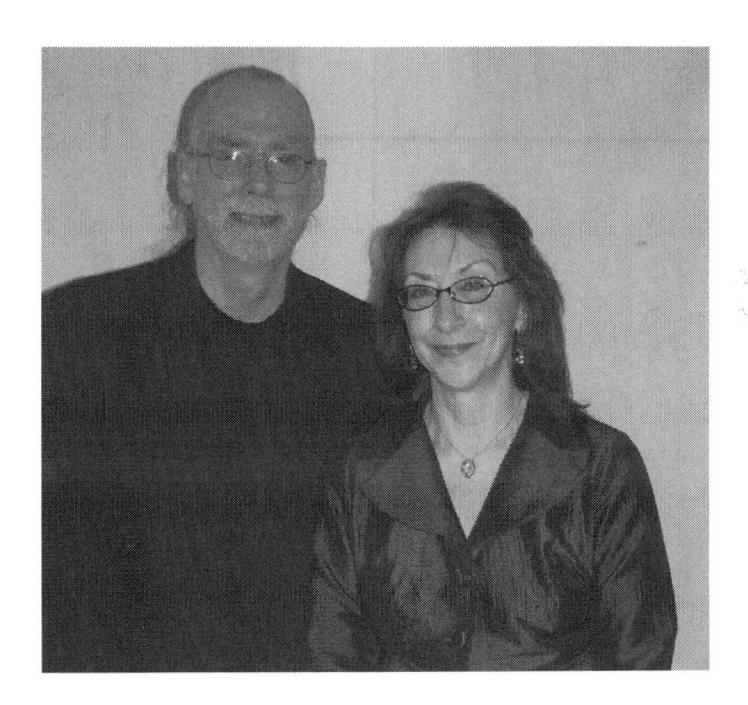

D*r. V. R. (Brick) Saunderson and his wife, Mona Saunderson, are clinical counseling hypnotherapists and co-owners of the CrossRoads Counselling Group in Parksville, Vancouver Island, British Columbia. Their*

twenty-plus-year practice is multidisciplinary and includes Reiki, acupressure, and cognitive therapy.

The following quotes were provided by Dr. Saunderson on August 23, 2012. We thank both Dr. Brick and Mona for their contribution to the section on hypnotherapy.

Introduction

Unlike many of the practitioners we have interviewed, Dr. Saunderson's journey to become a healer could not have been anticipated based on his early career choice. He started out as a town planner and was one of the founding members of the Association of Architectural Technologists in Ontario. And then he met Mona.

Dr. Saunderson describes Mona at the time of their meeting as a "new Christian," and it was within this context and through her wisdom that Dr. Saunderson began his own faith journey. Eventually, his understanding of faith took him into pastoral ministry. For fifteen years the Saundersons were engaged in pastoral ministry, setting up skilled-helper protocols within the ministry and teaching church elders skills such as empathy, immediacy, challenge, and so on. Their lives have been devoted to helping, teaching, and healing.

The Saundersons are travelers in life, ever learning along their journey, and what they discovered from their years in ministry is best explained by Dr. Saunderson:

> ...what we discovered ...what people needed most was to be heard...to be supported, cared for in a spirit without judgment...that everyone has value...there is no right, wrong, good, or bad; there is only the person's journey, and that journey is what is really important.

When they decided to leave the ministry, they made a natural transition to counseling and continued their process of discovery and lifelong learning. Soon they realized that while they were dealing with the emotional side of human beings, they were overlooking the physical aspect. As Dr. Saunderson explains it, "Because all the emotions that we experience manifest in our bodies, the entire body is an emotional being."

As a result of this understanding, they added bodywork to their practice and completed training and certification in acupressure and Reiki at the master's level. Therefore, when clients come to their clinic, Dr. Saunderson and his wife are not simply working with the cognitive and emotional aspects of the person's issue; they are also working with the way in which the person's life challenges are being physically embodied. "Our journey as healers", Dr. Saunderson states, "is a journey of looking at the needs of people and supporting people in their journey of life with the realization that there is no wrong journey. There is only the journey that you choose to take. Our job is to help people accomplish what they want to accomplish. That's it in a nutshell."

One can easily see that the Saundersons are multimodal practitioners and extraordinary teacher-healers, but for the purposes of this section, the Saundersons' skills and abilities as registered clinical counseling hypnotherapists are highlighted.

What Is Clinical Hypnotherapy?

To appreciate hypnotherapy, it is useful to have an understanding of hypnosis. Many people fear hypnosis, having developed an incorrect perception of the practice via religious, television, stage, and movie portrayals of hypnosis as a mysterious and compelling form of mind control. Nothing could be further from the truth. In truth, hypnosis is a natural phenomenon of the human mind. Dr. Saunderson explains:

> We all go in and out of hypnosis many times a day. We go into hypnosis automatically when we are reading,

when we're driving, [when we're] watching TV. An example that I often use is...have you ever gone to a movie...and the heroine dies and you're sitting there crying? I say, "Why are you crying? It's just a movie." But the mind cannot discern between reality and fantasy. And, as you are transfixed on the film, you enter into the experience as if it's real. You go into an altered state where you experience all the emotions as if they are really happening. That's hypnosis.

Although a hypnotherapist assists an individual to enter into an altered state of consciousness, with training a person is capable of entering into a hypnotic state simply referred to as self-hypnosis. All hypnosis is self-hypnosis. So when a client requests help from a professionally trained hypnotherapist to better manage personal and professional issues, she is asking for guidance through her own journey of self-hypnosis.

This means that the process of hypnotherapy is a relationship with a client who cannot presently meet his own needs out of his own resources[12]. At the request of the client, a hypnotherapist provides a skill-based service that is undertaken while a client is hypnotized. Hypnotherapy involves the use of several techniques, including using words and phrases to help clients navigate through life challenges. According to the glossary provided by the CrossRoads Training Institute (CRTI), hypnotherapy is "The treatment of any harmful, destructive or unwanted condition, mental or physical using hypnotism, and hypnotherapeutic suggestions"[13]. Pain, as an unwanted condition, is especially responsive to hypnotherapy.

---

12 Brick Saunderson, *CrossRoads Training Institute Manual (2010)*. Program Introduction: The Professional Hypnotist. Session 101, (Parksville, BC: CrossRoads Counselling Group).

13 Brick Saunderson, *CrossRoads Training Institute Manual (2010)*. A Glossary of Terms. (Parksville, BC: CrossRoads Counselling Group) 5.

What Causes Neck Soreness from a Hypnotherapy View?

Hypnotherapy is interested in pain as a total-person experience with many causes. Knowing that our bodies harbor emotional and spiritual pain within the physical is an important insight because the implication for the role of our minds in a pain experience is enormous. Hypnotherapy addresses the mind-body connection and the power of our thoughts in a critical way. Dr. Saunderson discusses how the way we talk about our pain can actually increase or decrease our pain level.

> As hypnotherapists, we never use the word *pain* because pain has a trigger mechanism just from the utilization of the word. So we never use it. When people come with pain, what we do is immediately reframe it as "discomfort." We're always talking about discomfort. The client may use the word *pain*, and we will reframe it back to him or her as discomfort: "Tell me about the discomfort that you're feeling."
>
> We have clients communicate their pain experience and scale it from one to ten and have them describe it... is it sharp, jagged, and so forth. They describe to us the sensation that the body is communicating. Then, we reframe it. Because we have the ability in our minds to actually change how we interpret the signal...if you're really, really good at it, [you can] actually block the signal from being communicated to the body.

Hypnotherapists can also have the brain reinterpret [pain] in some other way. There are techniques that they use to teach the client to manage the sensation of pain. So pain is a physical signal that is interpreted emotionally that they teach their clients to manage.

Differences between Men and Women

In the Saundersons' experience, men are more susceptible to a negative pain experience than are women. However, the ability to manage pain may be related to how much pain a person has endured so far in his or her life. Those who have lived with much pain may be less willing to tolerate more. One's response to pain is an individual, all-encompassing response based on experience and other stress-related factors.

The good news for adults with neck pain is that age and experience can prove to be an advantage to success with hypnotherapy. Dr. Saunderson explains:

> What is really fascinating is that older adults seem to have a stronger ability to let go. They are usually not as resistant. They're not as concerned. They really have a great desire to be helped, and so they are much more willing to give up control.
>
> Our experience with the older population, people fifty and over, is that they are much more capable of utilizing self-hypnosis. The older you are, the more wisdom you have and the more you are able to utilize hypnosis.

In terms of therapy, the differences are not so much gender-relevant as focused on differences within each individual. Each person has his own hypnotic talent. Because we are all unique, some of us more easily enter a trance state. Some of us can relax more easily; some of us trust more readily. Because we are different, we respond to different words and phrases. A skilled hypnotherapist will be aware of your needs and design therapy accordingly.

What You Can Expect When You Visit a Hypnotherapist

A hypnotherapist who is also trained in clinical counseling will be more highly skilled to work with your particular challenge.

Dr. Saunderson offers additional advice when considering hypnotherapy as a treatment for your pain:

> You want to ask first and foremost what the hypnotherapist's certification level is. For example, my wife and I are both registered clinical counseling hypnotherapists with the Association of Registered Clinical Hypnotherapists (ARCH) of Canada. You'll also find hypnotherapists who are members of the International Medical and Dental Hypnotherapy Association (IMDHA) in the United States. You want to look at what credentials a hypnotherapist carries. Other questions I would also ask are whether they are carrying professional liability insurance and how many hours of training they have. Also I would ask if they have knowledge in the area of your need. If, for example, I was going to someone for pain management, I would want to know what experience he had. So you would check him out as you would any therapist.

Once you have chosen a hypnotherapist, at your first visit, your hypnotherapist will complete a history of your medical conditions, life challenges, and current stressors. He will want to know your story—your family relationships, friendships, career path, employment and retirement experiences, and spiritual considerations. Because the history is so comprehensive, your hypnotherapist may even send you forms to complete prior to your first visit. Knowing who you are, what you are feeling, and how you think is important for successful treatment.

There are some restraints in the use of hypnotherapy. Mental illness associated with psychotic episodes and hallucinations is contraindicated because being in a hypnotic state places a susceptible person at risk for a further psychotic episode. If a client is under the influence of alcohol, drugs, or other substances, hypnosis is also not advised. In contrast, depression and anxiety respond well to hypnotherapy.

Understanding your pain history is also important. Your therapist will be taking note of the words and phrases that you use in the picture of life that you paint with your language. He may ask you to complete an assessment that will inform him about how you communicate and how you learn—whether you are a visual, auditory, or kinetic learner. Asking questions is encouraged and valued.

A discussion about hypnosis—what you understand about it and a full explanation of hypnosis and the hypnotic process—will help to relieve any anxiety that you may be experiencing. Finally, because hypnosis is so difficult to describe, expect to be provided with a sample of the hypnotic experience, which will put you even more at ease. Generally, the real work gets started with your second visit.

A hypnotherapist cannot hypnotize you without your permission. Remember that all hypnosis is self-hypnosis, so what you are doing is providing your readiness to partner with your hypnotherapist to relieve your pain. Therefore, the second visit sets the stage for your first encounter with hypnosis. One technique that can be used to address your pain is called the color technique. Dr. Saunderson explains it as such:

> The therapist has the client give the pain a color, a shape, and a size, and then asks the client to change the color, shape, and size in his mind....For example, we may say, "Give the discomfort a color, and he may say "red"...and then you ask him, "What is your favorite color?" and he may say "blue." Then we say, "OK, change the color from red to blue." All of a sudden, just by changing the color, you've changed how that sensation manifests in his mind.

Another part of this technique emphasizes the size of the client's pain. When asked about the size of his or her pain, Dr. Saunders continues, the client may liken it to a "basketball."

> Then you say, "Reduce it to the size of a pea." And she can mentally make that discomfort get smaller and

smaller and smaller. Obviously, this technique takes practice. Some people are really proficient at it, and they can change the sensation immediately. Others take a little bit more practice to really master this.

Many people can visualize objects, memories, colors, and so forth. Likewise many cannot. People who have difficulty visualizing probably are more sensitive to sounds or words that convey feelings such as soft, rough, prickly, and so on. You and your hypnotherapist partner to determine your perceptual strengths. In this way, you will gain the greatest benefit from hypnosis.

Partnering with Your Hypnotherapist

Learning how to manage your own pain is the ultimate goal of hypnotherapy. In this regard, you are in a mentor-student relationship, where each has a responsibility to the other in order to help you achieve pain relief.

Your responsibility is to ask questions, provide information, practice the relaxation techniques or other homework provided, and keep an open mind when being introduced to new information. Your therapist's role is to help you become independent by increasing your capacity to monitor and manage your pain. As Dr. Saunderson states, "Pain management is about teaching clients to self-care; that is the first priority." Learning to relax your body and mind through self-hypnosis frees, empowers, and enables you to live your life more fully, more vibrantly.

> When a person is able to relax, to physically relax his body and mentally relax the mind, what he will immediately discover is the reduction of any kind of discomfort—as much as 75 percent....Most of the pain we experience in our physical bodies we actually accentuate by trying not to suffer....We do that by putting our body in various

positions; we tighten our muscles, and that acts as an amplifier of discomfort. The things that we're trying to do to avoid pain are actually making the pain worse. So, one of the great gifts of hypnosis is relaxation of the physical and emotional self.

In partnership with your hypnotherapist, you have an opportunity to become more aware of yourself—how you think about and respond to life. Perhaps more than any other therapy, hypnotherapy raises awareness about the power of the mind-body connection and the value of the placebo effect.

What Is Reiki?

Because the Saundersons are holistic healers whose practice involves work with the mind and body simultaneously, we decided to include an explanation of one of their other treatment modalities—Reiki.

> The word Reiki (pronounced ray-key) is a Japanese kanji for universal life-force energy...Reiki is simple and produces measurable results...It is power, light, and love. Reiki transcends the man-made divisions of religion, economics, location, gender, and race.[14]

Although Reiki involves the use of the practitioner's hands, it is not massage therapy. Reiki works with your body's unique energy and is used in conjunction with medical and complementary treatments. Generally, Reiki is a spiritually based practice in that it trusts the body to heal itself and works well when mending stress-

---

14 Canadian Reiki Association, "About Reiki-FAQS," *What is the Usui System of Natural Healing?*, http://www.reiki.ca/faqs.htm#6 (accessed 39 Aug. 2012)

related conditions[15]. As the client, you recline upon a treatment or massage table and remain fully clothed. After a discussion of your specific health issue, neck pain, the Reiki practitioner will use his hands positioned four to six inches above your body to move and unblock your body's vital energy. You will likely experience a feeling of warmth, relaxation, and calm. Some people have a tingling sensation as their energy is moved and balanced through the art and practice of a skilled Reiki therapist. Other Reiki therapies include therapeutic touch, healing hands, and the laying on of hands. Reiki is used in hospitals, multidisciplinary clinics, and private practices all over the globe.

Conclusion

A clinical counseling hypnotherapist helps clients use their minds to influence their bodies. In this way, clinical hypnotherapy honors the bodymind as a whole, not the body and mind as separate entities. Working on the body and mind simultaneously has a real advantage in pain management. Moreover, with the goal of helping you, the client, master self-hypnosis, clinical hypnotherapy is an empowering collaborative strategy for total pain management. Once learned, self-hypnosis spills over into other areas of your life, relieving stress and centering you so that life is far more enjoyable.

---

15 Pamela Miles, "Reiki, Medicine and Self Care with Pamela Miles," *Reiki, Spiritual Practice or Energy Medicine?* http://reikiinmedicine.org/healthful-lifestyle/reiki-practice-energy-med/ (accessed 31 Aug. 2012).

Chapter Nine: Integrative Nutrition and Health Counselor

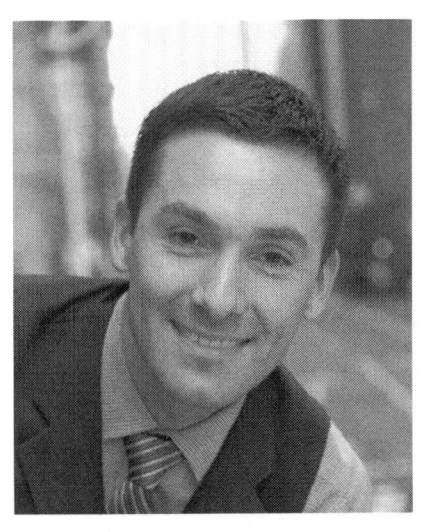

Patrick Martin Jr. is an integrative and holistic health counselor in private practice since 2008 at Northwest Integrative Wellness in the greater Seattle area of Washington State. He holds diplomas from the Institute for Integrative Nutrition and from the Teachers College at Columbia University. Some of his teachers include Dr. Andrew Weil, director of the Arizona Center for Integrative Medicine, and Dr. Deepak Chopra, leader in the field of mind-body medicine.

The following quotes were provided by Patrick Martin Jr. on August 27, 2012. We thank Patrick for his contribution to the section on integrative nutrition and health counselor.

Introduction

Patrick has had a truly challenging journey to find the fit between who he is and what he does. From the age of nine until his twenties, Patrick suffered from serious health challenges. His challenges were so severe that in his late teens he weighed 270 pounds, was deemed permanently disabled, and was awarded social supplementary income and medical coverage. Patrick explains his lowest point:

> In the late nineties, it was believed that I would never go to school or work again. I couldn't hold my focus for longer than five, maybe ten, seconds. I was a mess physically and mentally. Basically, it was believed that the rest of my life was going to be spent recycling into the health-care system to treat all of the conditions I had been diagnosed with.

Fortunately for Patrick, help was not far away. By happenstance, it became necessary for Patrick to change therapists. He chose an individual in a neighboring town and thus began his journey of recovery. Although his new therapist was providing counseling services, he also had a background in holistic health care. Patrick describes his experience with this therapist, whom he calls "one of the most influential people in my shift toward healthier living."

> He told me that if I could help it, to not eat anything with a label, ever. If it grows in nature, it is a whole food, and it is OK to go ahead and eat it as long as my body agrees with it. If you do eat something with a label, make sure that you can pronounce everything on the label and understand what the ingredients are. If you think about it, there are no maltodextrin bushes or polysaccharide trees. These are processed things that have vital components stripped from them, and therefore we should not put them into our bodies. If we do eat them, our bodies are going to respond accordingly: junk in, junk out.

From these first insights about the significance that food choice has in good health, Patrick began a journey of self-discovery. Over the next couple of years, Patrick found a Reiki teacher who advised him to also remove wheat from his diet and to keep track of any changes he noticed in a journal. Knowing that a journey into self-discovery requires an open mind and a willingness to try new approaches, Patrick followed her instructions.

> At first I didn't notice anything, and I thought, OK, this is strange. When I reintroduced the wheat products into my diet, I completely decompensated psychologically and became delusional and paranoid, and I encountered states of anxiety bordering on what is considered a panic attack, which were only a few of the symptoms I had struggled with when I was growing up. So I removed wheat from my diet and started a gluten-free lifestyle.

The gluten-free diet made such a dramatic difference in the way Patrick felt that it actually inspired his decision to launch a career as an integrative nutrition and health counselor. "From that point on," Patrick recalls, "I really became interested in the effect that food has on the mind, the body, and the spirit."

As he began his studies, Patrick was led to another mentor, and together they discovered that since early childhood, Patrick had been suffering the accumulating effects of mercury amalgam fillings. Laboratory tests showed that Patrick had high levels of mercury in his system, and it was determined that he was living with what was considered a mild form of mercury exposure. Eventually he found a holistic dentist who extracted all of his amalgam and replaced it with a compound that was nontoxic to his body. Other aspects of his therapy included chelation and nutritional therapy supervised by a naturopathic physician who specialized in biochemical individuality and nutrition. Within two months, he was taken off all medication and was symptom-free. He has remained free of medication and symptoms for the past fifteen years.

Patrick finally had his health and his life back, and as a young man in his early twenties, he was ready to reclaim his future.

> I petitioned the court and had the disability judgment reversed, and I enrolled in school. That was the beginning of my journey to rebuild my education and to build a career path. I knew that I wanted to do something in regard to healing and working with people who had mental illnesses as well as other health conditions....I knew that I wanted my career path to focus on integrating something about nutrition and its healing effects....I started as a psychology major, earning an associate's degree in human services and a bachelor's degree in the humanities. During the latter is when I found the Institute for Integrative Nutrition.

What Is Integrative Health Counseling?

Integrative health counseling is a holistic health-care practice that helps clients become aware of and resolve problems in key areas in their lives in order to return to health. Key areas for consideration include relationships, career, spirituality, and exercise. While the client undertakes intensive work in these key areas the integrative health counselor will be slowly and systematically introducing his client to healthy, whole foods that are natural, organic, and frequently locally grown. In this way, integrative health counseling is all-inclusive, attending to body, mind, and spirit.

> Beyond food, other forms of nourishment—what our school calls primary foods—are essential for health. A spiritual practice, a desired career, regular physical activity, and healthy relationships fill your soul and satisfy your hunger for living. When primary food is balanced and fulfilling, the fun, excitement, and passion of your daily life feed you.[16]

---

16 Faculty Integrative Nutrition Institute, and Robin Peglow. *The Integrative Nutrition Journal.* (New York: Integrative Nutrition Publishing, 2006). 1

What Causes Neck Soreness from an Integrative Health Counseling View?

As we age, diet, environmental stressors, and hormonal changes lead to low levels of inflammation in our bodies. Over time, this kind of low-grade inflammation begins to take its toll on our health. Most chronic diseases associated with aging (e.g., arthritis, heart disease, and diabetes) result from inflammation. Patrick advises, "While movement is a vital tool, it serves only as a temporary solution to a systemic issue." Patrick further explains:

> Toxins in the body are a significant culprit in many cases of soreness and inflammation in all ages; this is oftentimes seen in people who have pollution-induced toxicity. Think contaminated air, water, and food sources, as well as heavy metals from amalgam fillings, and the like. Because the body is not able to effectively rid itself of the toxin as it would in minimal exposures, the body thinks that it is constantly being invaded. Consequently, the immune system activates and fights the invaders [toxins] and does not shut down because there is a constant stream of toxins from the air, water, food, and so forth.
>
> Eventually, the immune system begins to break down the body as seen in autoimmune disease. Think of it as glowing embers in a fire that are smoldering very slowly. That low burn is akin to the inflammation we see in the body of [the elderly]. The idea is to help the individual add appropriate practices and foods into his life that are going to extinguish or cool that fire.

The food choices that we make as we age can either contribute to continued inflammation or work to reduce it. Foods that create and perpetuate inflammation are those that are processed and high in sugars and starches, such as baked goods, pastries, pasta, and snack foods. The release of sugar into our bloodstream as a consequence of eating these foods produces the pro-inflammatory response. Inflammation is also destructive to tissue, causing pain, stiffness, and swelling in muscles and joints, and as such contributes significantly to an experience of neck pain and discomfort.

The aches and pains we feel as we age are not always related to arthritis: they may actually be a signal from the body that changes in diet, exercise, and relationships are needed[17]. And these aches and pains that we believe are normal may be more pronounced today than in years past. Patrick explains this phenomenon:

> Seniors of today did not start their lives with processed foods. When seniors were children, their bodies were raised on wholesome, nutritious foods. They didn't have these boxed foods; they didn't have all these sugar-laden foods on a daily basis. They had whole foods that were probably grown within ten miles of where they were living, if not on their own farm. They were connected to the earth. They were raised healthy, their food was healthy, and their communities were healthy. I think that's something that has been lost.

When one considers the other major changes in society, including technological innovation, the inundation and intrusion of the media in our information-driven world, and the challenge of air and water pollution, one begins to understand the impact of stressors in the lives of today's seniors. Today's lifestyle can seem foreign and out of sync to elders raised in a different time, and their state of health is a warning red flag about their inability to adapt.

Differences between Men and Women

Patrick believes that the only differences between male and female clients are age-related hormonal changes. Hormonal changes in

---

17 Organic Excellence, "Alternative Joint Pain Therapies," http://www.organicexcellence.com/we-alternative_joint_pain_therapies.php (accessed 8 Sept. 2012),

women begin at menopause, when estrogen production begins to decline. In men, andropause—the gradual reduction of testosterone levels—begins in middle age. For men, the hormonal changes occur at a slower pace than for women. Depletion in hormones can lead to osteoporosis and can ultimately cause loss of bone resulting in potential fractures and neck pain.

Factors other than gender play a larger role in the differences Patrick sees among his clients. Most important is one's unique biological and biochemical makeup. He explains how he addresses this difference:

> Not everybody responds to chiropractic, homeopathic remedy, qigong exercises, or acupuncture in the same way....I'm not a fan of cookie-cutter approaches to wellness, and so I think that each individual requires a specific configuration of tools, tailored to her individual needs (exercise, foods, spiritual practices, and the like), that will assist her healing process...every single detail that makes that person who she is—her history, her ancestral heritage, even her blood type.

Although important, we are more than the sum of our biological material. Research has found that, through our intentions, we can change our DNA. In studies conducted at the Institute of HeartMath, scientists found that the research data related to one's intention to adopt a positive attitude, "indicate that when individuals are in a heart-focused, loving state and in a more coherent mode of physiological functioning, they have a greater ability to alter the conformation (shape or structure) of DNA.[18]" Adopting and maintaining a positive attitude can directly affect overall health. Meditation, yoga, quiet walks, counseling and any number of

---

18 Institute of HeartMath, "Emotions Can Change Your DNA." *Newsletter Vol. 11/No 4,* (Winter 2012), http://www.heartmath.org/templates/ihm/e-newsletter/publication/2012/winter/emotions-can-change-your-dna.php?mtcCampaign=22257&mtcEmail=98739165 (accessed 13 Dec. 2012),

activities that help us reframe our experiences and maintain an optimistic outlook have the same effect.

What You Can Expect When You Visit an Integrative Health Counselor

When you visit an integrative health counselor, be prepared for a complete, total-person assessment; integrative health counselors believe that whatever is happening in your life is expressed in the state of your health. Patrick explains a typical first visit:

> When I bring somebody in, I do a health assessment with him. It's a little bit different from most assessments in that we focus on several areas that most people in nutrition do not focus on—we get to know each other on a deep level, in a safe, nonjudgmental client-provider relationship. We explore the client's relationships, career/retirement path, spiritual health, exercise, what sort of resources he has available to him, and so on. All of these different components, as well as many subcategories, go into how a treatment plan will be designed for the specific needs of the client.

Patrick completes such a comprehensive history for each client's treatment plan because he recognizes the complex and individual nature of each person who seeks his help. A typical treatment plan is designed to cover a six-month period because, according to experts in the field of integrative health, that's how long it takes a person to change old habits and reinforce new ones.

A substantial part of the treatment begins with detoxification to clear the body of vitality-robbing toxins. Detoxification—removing impurities from the body by resting, fasting, and replenishing the body with nutrients—serves to enhance immune system function, improve cell wall function, and restore the body to its natural balance. Further reduction of the inflammatory process involves, for some, the use of nutrigenomics, which Patrick defines as a *"field of functional medicine that uses nutrition to alter gene expression in the body."* In other words, nutrigenomics focus on the relationship between your diet and your genes with the aim to personalize your nutrient intake.

Patrick uses nutriceuticals, which are food-based supplements and medical foods used for management of chronic disease. He also uses nutritional supplements, omega-3 oils, and fish oils, along with other dietary changes and exercise programs, to assist his clients' shift back to health.

Partnering with Your Integrative Health Counselor

During the course of the six-month program, you will likely be required to meet with your integrative health counselor every two weeks. In addition, you will be asked to complete homework assignments between sessions. Learning is focused on not only changing your dietary habits but also changing your relationship to food, including how you, the client, have been using food in your life. Thus journaling is also a core component of the program because learning comes from reflection on our motivations and behaviors—what we choose to eat and why we choose it.

Patrick outlines two common homework assignments:

> In client sessions, I give my clients tools such as cookbooks. When they receive the book, I also give them a variety of different greens, grains, or protein samples, and I'll have them select a variety of recipes to try. Initially their homework will be to integrate those recipes into their lives within the next week or two weeks between sessions to keep them actively engaged in the transition process.
>
> I also have them go into the community where they shop. I have them pay attention to what they see—how foods are marketed, how markets are arranged, how the

marketing is affecting their decisions, what other people are putting into their carts. I want to cultivate a sense of awareness around food and what influences their decisions to purchase certain foods and how they can avoid that or work with that to make better choices.

Reflection on the quality of one's relationships is also a key to learning new behaviors. Engaging in conversations with your integrative health counselor about spiritual concerns and social and family issues is important for growth in self-knowledge and self-awareness, as well as for identifying underlying causes for poor lifestyle choices. Patrick believes:

There's a big disconnect in people's understanding of how relationships affect their health...if you have somebody who's in a relationship that is not nurturing or sustaining, then the effect that it can have on [his or her] body is profound, and vice versa. I support my clients in identifying and securing nourishing and sustaining relationships and activities.

Relational discord and conflict within families, friendships, and communities can lead to disharmony expressed through health-risk behaviors. In an attempt to reduce stress and anxiety, people may engage in emotional eating, compulsive shopping, gambling, and other addictive behaviors with alcohol or drugs. However, a single nurturing, sustaining relationship with another trusted person can turn those behaviors around. This is the reason for continual evaluation of our lives in the context of others and their effect upon us.

Retirement, which can lead to loss of connection, loss of meaning, loneliness, and isolation, may also put older adults at risk. Your partnership with your integrative health counselor is one relationship. Volunteering, joining in social activities, or joining a senior citizen group can help one avert a retirement without meaning. Becoming more spiritually aware or becoming part of a faith community is another way to find nurturance and meaning. When our connections are invested in positive supports, we are empowered. We grow in confidence; we have more energy and need to rely less on old habits.

All of these facets of one's life are examined with an integrative health counselor because the experience of pain is a total-person experience. Therefore, the best approach to relieving pain and discomfort requires a total-person assessment and treatment plan.

Continual evaluation over the six-month period is essential to ensure that clients understand and have incorporated the changes that Patrick has been teaching them. A large number of the lifestyle changes can be attributed to client education. Integrative health counselors are at heart change agents, and education is at the root of change. Careful observation and education are important factors in the client-counselor partnership.

Conclusion

Integrative nutritional counselors understand that we feed ourselves in many ways—through our relationships, careers, family histories, education, and more. In his practice, Patrick has demonstrated the multiple ways in which an integrative nutritionist can partner with you to address your pain experience from multiple perspectives; but, always with a keen awareness of the critical role that nutrition plays.

It is also important to take into consideration the fact that many of us use food for reasons other than hunger. Eating is linked to relationship issues. Because humans are social, we need to develop self-awareness and understanding in terms of ourselves, our families, and our social worlds. The quality of our relationships with others, with ourselves, and with our creator can either support or damage our health. Although the choice is ours, an integrative health counselor can assist with your choices.

Chapter Ten: Pilates

*E*rica Trokey is a chiropractor and a Pilates program teacher and coach in St. Charles, Missouri. Currently, she owns and instructs at her own studio, Trokey Pilates Studio in New Town at St. Charles.

The following quotes are Dr. Trokey's provided on August 8, 2012. We thank Dr. Trokey for her contribution to the following section on Pilates.

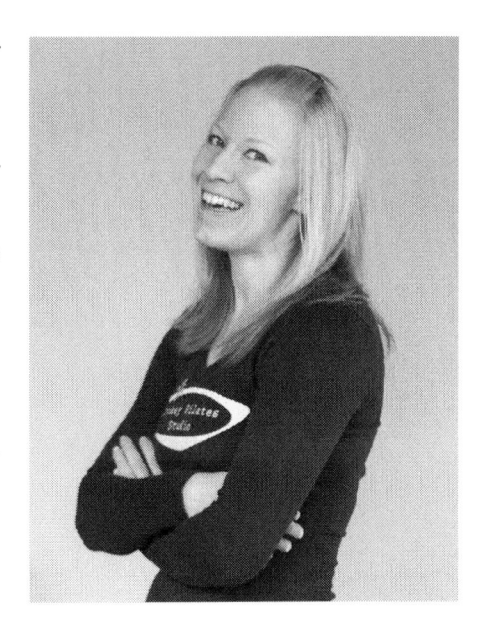

Introduction

Always interested in science, Dr. Trokey easily gravitated toward the health and human sciences. However, two life-changing events shaped her final decision to establish a career in health care. The first significant event involved a back injury from a fall. The second involved a sports injury incurred while lifting weights. Each of her injuries led to chiropractic care and an ensuing interest in the field of health and wellness. After spending one hour a day working in her chiropractor's office as part of her educational program in senior high school, her decision was made. She committed to continuing her education and earned her bachelor's degree in human biology and, eventually, her doctorate in chiropractic medicine.

During her studies in chiropractic college, she began taking Pilates classes to keep her body fit while she exercised her mind. She "loved Pilates" and continued to pursue her practice of Pilates over the following ten years. When it came time for her to make a career shift, her love of Pilates made her decision easy. She completed her Pilates training via Balanced Body®, one of the largest facilities for Pilates education, and has "never looked back."

Dr. Trokey is unique in her preparation to teach Pilates in that she was originally trained in chiropractic. She has a profound understanding of human musculoskeletal structures and how they need to move for optimum health. Having owned and worked in two different pain clinics, she has many years' experience in a multispecialty team setting. Therefore, her years in chiropractic medicine and holistic health care inform both her Pilates practice and instruction.

What is Pilates?

Pilates is a program of exercise as opposed to a health-care therapy and, according to Dr. Trokey, is defined as "a form of exercise involving resistance, body alignment, core strength, and stabilization to help the body learn to perform at its greatest potential."

What Causes Neck Soreness from a Pilates View?

Falls, accidents, and injuries involving the neck, back, or shoulders at a young age can have serious consequences in older adults. As we age, the bones in our body tend to go through a process of degeneration that commonly includes the neck vertebrae and joint spaces of the cervical spine—the area of the spine that immediately supports our head.

Early trauma, even minor sports injuries or a simple fender bender, can cause micro tears in the ligaments that support and stabilize the bones of the neck. According to Dr. Trokey, such injuries set a painful process in motion:

> If you're not doing anything rehabilitative, then those neck bones are shifting and moving. Even a minor accident can cause abnormal motion or excess motion in the cervical spine. Once that starts to happen, the body is going to try to neutralize and control that motion. It's a natural reaction. The body wants to stabilize the neck by creating more bone. That's why people get bone spurs. The body will tend to try to fuse itself together to minimize that excess movement; that's how chronic conditions come about.

Where there is joint and vertebra involvement, there is also implication for a muscular response. Inflammation due to either recent injury or trauma much earlier in life causes the muscles of the neck and shoulders to respond by tensing. The tension can also result from emotional issues, relationships problems, financial challenges, and other concerns.

> The muscle tension that you experience comes from your trapezii (trap) muscles in your upper neck and shoulder area. As your trap muscles tighten, they trigger other muscles to contract. Muscle tension and tightening is indicative of muscles that are overworking to compensate for the smaller postural muscle groups that may

have shut down. The postural muscle groups should be working at all times to support and stabilize the neck. When the postural muscle groups fail to respond adequately, the larger muscles take over. When the large muscles such as your traps and rhomboids take over, you begin to experience trigger points and radiating pain, which in turn promote headaches and neck pain.

Headaches and painful trigger points along the neck and shoulders may indicate to you that it is time to think seriously about looking for a Pilates instructor because, as Dr. Trokey states, "It takes a lot of retraining to get those smaller postural muscle groups to start to activate again and to work in the way they were originally designed. Once they do work properly, those large muscle groups can stop constantly overworking."

As we age and we incur more neck and shoulder injuries, even if those injuries are minor, our chances of having chronic neck problems substantially increase. This is particularly true if such injuries remain untreated. Therefore, it is important to be aware of the seriousness of any upper-body injury, no matter how small. Better yet, by improving our overall muscle and joint conditioning through a Pilates program, we can improve balance and coordination and reduce the risk of accident and injury.

Pilates works on another level: the mind-body connection. Your brain and body are intimately connected and in continuous communication. When a health challenge becomes long-term and chronic, it indicates miscommunication between your brain and body. In neck problems, your muscles may have been continually activated and fired up over a long period, finally losing their capacity to relax. Being able to tell your muscles to relax and stay relaxed aids in reestablishing healthy mind-body communication. Pilates is geared toward making your brain aware of which muscles you are using and when you are using them—how they connect and engage.

Another aspect of the mind-body connection is found in the proprioceptive system necessary for coordination and balance. Dr. Trokey explains the connection in this way:

> Receptor nerves located in muscles, joints, and the ligaments around joints are what comprise this system. When injury occurs, the receptors become damaged and lose their ability to send messages to our brain. Consequently, our balance and coordination is affected. By working on the proprioceptive system, the communication between the brain and joints is improved, resulting in better muscle control, engagement, and awareness.

Coordination in an older population is hugely important because poor coordination can easily result in a fall. As long as the proprioceptive system is functioning and firing, seniors are less at risk for broken bones and damaged joints.

What You Can Expect When You Visit a Pilates Instructor

Originally, Pilates exercises were offered on a one-to-one basis, but they have moved to small groups or large classes. Nonetheless, for older adults who present with specific neck problems, the best approach remains individualized attention or membership in a very small group. Dr. Trotsky advises the following:

> If you're going for the therapy aspect to help with the chronic neck pain, you probably should stay away from a big gym environment and give yourself a private individual studio specific to Pilates where they focus in depth on Pilates and where the instructor is open to your communication.

The exercises and various movements you will be learning as a student of Pilates are usually performed in bare feet. If you find working out in bare feet uncomfortable, you can wear socks, but preferably those with nonslip soles. The body heat and perspiration you'll generate require that you dress very comfortably. Select clothing that is not only comfortable but also will fit in such a way as to allow your instructor to check your position, alignment, and the quality of your muscles' responses. Workout clothing can be purchased most anywhere as yoga, qigong, and other forms of exercise have become more popular for all ages. A whole new fashion industry has arisen around workout clothes. Clothes that are designed and manufactured for workouts avoid the use of zippers, buttons, and other fasteners, which can be very uncomfortable for mat work. Have fun: experiment with color and style. Why not try that hot pink outfit, expose those legs, and enjoy yourself?

Perfume and other scents (natural oils, lotions) are usually contraindicated at Pilates studios or gymnasiums. You will also want to avoid all but your most basic jewelry (wedding ring) because necklaces and bracelets could get damaged or become caught in Pilates equipment.

Pilates uses exercise mats as well as Pilates-specific equipment. One piece of equipment that looks rather daunting with its straps, springs, pulleys, and ropes is called a reformer. It is designed specifically to work with the principles and goals of Pilates, and it works in two important ways. First it provides resistance to work specific muscles and muscle groups, and second it assists clients through their exercise program by supporting individuals who have a limited range of motion to engage in modified exercises. Some reformers are wooden, and others are metal; some are raised up from the floor, and others sit flush. There is no age restriction for reformer usage. Clients of any age can safely use a reformer as long as they are able to get up and down from the reformer.

Partnering with Your Pilates Instructor

Dr. Trokey's background as a chiropractor enables her to take a more therapeutic look at her clients, but Pilates instructors come from many backgrounds, including physiotherapy, massage therapy, fitness training, and other health- and fitness-related industries. All are professionally trained in the Joseph Pilates method. Therefore, you can feel safe and confident when working with a Pilates instructor.

What is important to remember is that you, the student/client, are the center of interest for your Pilates instructor. Her role is to help you observe and understand the changes that are occurring and will occur in your muscle tone, balance, posture, and range of motion as you work through the program. But you must be prepared to do the work. A large part of your work is to be open to instructions and communicate with your instructor. She will need to know how you are feeling, whether or not you are experiencing pain beyond your comfort level, and if you have questions about the pace or design of your program.

Dr. Trokey is aware of the unique needs of an aging population as well as some of the challenges faced by older adults who are living with neck problems. In this regard she advises to, "keep your pace slower—do not rush from one neck exercise to the next." Also, "try to keep slow and controlled movements so that the brain really has time to think about what muscle is firing right now." Dr. Trokey teaches her clients to stay at a pace that is healthy for them and to avoid forcing their joints to move too quickly.

She notes the importance of communication concerning one's pain experience during the workout:

> I always tell my students, please communicate with me. If we're doing something in class and you're feeling pain, then it's not the type of thing that you should be doing. It's not a no-pain, no-gain atmosphere. If you're feeling something uncomfortable in your body, then that's not a good thing. Speak up; say something. We can modify your workout so that it's beneficial to your body.

Further, Dr. Trokey encourages her students to let her know about their pain or symptoms even after the class, in the days following the workout. Dr. Trokey believes that the Pilates exercises should be helpful, not hurtful. She emphasizes, "If an instructor keeps saying, 'Push through it; push through it,' that, in my opinion, is not Pilates." Rather, she is committed to a partnership between instructor and student in which both aim to benefit the body in a pain-free way.

If you find that your instructor is not open to ongoing communication with you or the class you are attending is too group focused and your needs are unmet, find a Pilates instructor who will work on a one-to-one basis with you. Being older and having long suffered with neck pain indicates that individual instruction is more appropriate for you.

Finally, partnership means developing healthy lifestyle habits between classes. There is one important activity that will enhance the work you're doing at your Pilates sessions: walking. Something as simple as developing a walking habit will help because movement keeps your blood flowing, nourishing your muscles and nerves as you walk. In this way, walking is great for the spine. When you're sedentary, there's no way for the nutrients that flow through the spinal column to get out to the nerves and keep them functioning at their optimum. And this communication between the brain and the body is essential.

Dr. Trokey advises against the use of soft collars for neck pain relief. She cautions if you are tempted to use a soft collar for neck support, your neck muscles may begin to rely on the collar, resulting in a loss of muscle tone and strength. Joints are meant to move, so moving your head and neck is a way to keep your muscles and joints healthy.

Some people who are experiencing post-exercise pain like to place a heated beanbag around their neck and shoulders. Heat can feel wonderful on a sore neck, but it can be detrimental. Applying heat can actually stimulate inflammation, which in turn causes more pain. Dr. Trokey cautions, "Heat can cause more harm than good. If you're going to use heat, then follow it with ice." The next chapter on physiotherapy (under the section Ways to Manage a Painful Episode) will provide additional information for reducing pain and inflammation.

Conclusion

Pilates is a program rather than a therapy. Joseph Pilates, its founder, developed his unique exercise program to improve strength, flexibility, body coordination, and range of motion for all the different joints and muscles within the human body. Working one-on-one with an instructor specifically trained in Pilates can greatly improve your body's functional ability as well as enhance your sense of well-being. It can also reduce your pain and introduce you to a new activity that can be fun.

Chapter Eleven: Physiotherapy

Ernest Ball is a physiotherapist who has a special interest in rehabilitation and sports medicine. He is the owner of the Cumbria Physiotherapy Clinic in Qualicum Beach on Vancouver Island, British Columbia, Canada.

The following quotes were provided by Ernest on August 28, 2012. We thank Ernest for his contribution to the section on physiotherapy.

Introduction

From an early age, Ernie was interested in how the body functioned. In his late teens, he started practicing the Japanese martial art of aikido. It is a holistic practice, combining martial art studies, philosophy, and spirituality. Ernie has been teaching the art of aikido for the past forty-five years, and it was his early discipline and training in the art that eventually led him to a career in physical medicine. Ernie explains the influence of aikido on his life's work:

> One of the features of practicing and teaching aikido is you learn a lot about your body and about other people's bodies...you have to watch them and carefully grade everything. So you begin to develop body awareness. That was the start for me—teaching people, seeing them improve, seeing them get stronger, move better, and perform the techniques. I felt I really wanted to do something worthwhile and not just do an average job. Basically I just wanted to make a difference...I really had that call.

As with other health-care professionals who obtain great pleasure from helping people back to health, for Ernie the work of physical medicine is a gratifying experience.

> To care for a person with severe trauma, perhaps in intensive care, then see them progress to a ward and eventually return home, then treating them as an outpatient and finally enabling them to return to work is a fantastic thing. This is what I felt I was called to do.

What Is Physiotherapy?

The Physiotherapy Foundation of Canada (PFC) describes physiotherapy as a "health care profession directed at evaluating, restoring and maintaining physical function.[19]" The ability to fulfill the mandate of the PFC requires highly trained professionals, and the required level of education and training continues to grow with new knowledge and technologies in health care. Because of its medical science basis, physiotherapy is more a part of conventional medicine than all other therapies presented. It

---

19 Physiotherapy Foundation of Canada, "What is Physiotherapy?" http://www.physiotherapyfoundation.ca/about_what_is_physiotherapy.html (accessed 3 Sept. 2012).

is also holistic in its approach to client care and very valuable in the management of neck pain. Ernie furthers our understanding with his own definition:

> Physiotherapists study the human body in all its aspects: anatomy, physiology, neurology—all the body systems—in addition to arthrokinematics [how joints move] and kinesiology [the way we move]. For example, when we perform research, we have to be able to measure performance and movement and assess any impairment or dysfunction in the patient. This even applies to respiratory function or any specific joint in the body. Our aim is to restore function, to rehabilitate. Physiotherapy treatment is a process. We have to be able to motivate and encourage the patient to participate and work through what may be in some cases a painful and distressing period.

What Causes Neck Soreness from a Physiotherapy View?

According to physiotherapists, there are several causes for chronic neck pain in older adulthood. One of the most prevalent is postural change over a lifetime. Ernie explains why these postural changes occur:

> This can be brought about by inactivity or by a lifetime of work habits over many years. Other causes are degenerative changes in the spine, in this case the neck, the bones, joints, and soft tissue of the upper back. Inactivity can also play a major role; for example, retirement may cause someone to become suddenly less active.

Psychosocial issues may also contribute to inactivity in an older person. We can feel overwhelming sadness, lack of energy, and disinterest in socializing because of losses like the death of a spouse, family member, or friend. Poor adaptation to retirement can also leave us housebound. Ernie explains, "When we're depressed, we may not go out as much. We may find it difficult to be active, so we develop postural issues."

In addition, old injuries such as dislocations and fractures caused by falls, motor vehicle accidents, and sports can contribute to spine and joint problems as we age. Having attended many clients with such injuries, Ernie advises:

> You don't have to be in a vehicle to get a whiplash injury. For example, if you stumble over a rock on the beach but you don't fall, you can jar your neck enough to cause pain. In an older person, this can cause a whiplash effect. Falls are another thing that can jar the neck. Sometimes a jarring motion can even cause a fracture in someone with any underlying disease that affects the strength of the bones.

There may also be underlying disease processes that cause inflammation, weaken the bones, or make them more brittle, such as osteoarthritis, osteoporosis, and cancer. Long-term use of steroid medications can adversely affect the strength of bones and soft tissue as well.

Neck pain can be caused by the effects of osteoarthritis, whereby the cartilage that lines the joints becomes worn and inflamed and often bone spurs form. Sometimes the degeneration in our bones, joints, and soft tissue in the absence of a disease process, is a part of the natural process of aging. The general wear and tear of a long life has a damaging effect on our bones and joints.

Physiotherapists are trained to evaluate the presence or severity of arthritis by physical examination. In other words, X-rays may not always tell the whole story. "In terms of the spine," Ernie explains, "you may have a person with an X-ray showing lots of arthritis who may be symptom-free. Conversely, the opposite is often true."

Have you become shorter as you age? Loss of height occurs because the discs between your vertebrae become worn down. They also become dehydrated. When discs lose their ability to cushion vertebrae, the sensation of bone rubbing against bone can be very painful. In both instances, the discs may lose much of their ability to absorb shock as they become thinner and harder. In addition to pain, some people may also appear to shrink as they age.

Differences between Men and Women

As men and women age, the effects of aging may differ, mainly due to body strength and the effects of their previous work life. Men are more likely to have had a more physical occupation. Their experiences of pain may also be different. Women may often do more repetitive duties and chores throughout their lives. Ernie explains the difference from a physiotherapist's perspective:

> The lady of the house usually continues her usual household duties, depending on the age, of course—doing the housework, doing the cooking....but housework can be challenging because it involves a lot of bending, a lot of head-forward postures, a lot of pulling and pushing, vacuum cleaning, sweeping, picking things up...groceries. All of these things may contribute to neck, upper-back, or shoulder pain.

Ernie continues that men, on the other hand, may have fewer daily chores of the repetitive kind but tend to have heavier work, such as "carrying the ladder, putting it up, climbing up, and reaching.... lifting things, mowing the lawn, digging, making things, or performing construction around the house and yard."

What to Expect When You Visit a Physiotherapist

Physiotherapists, like all holistic practitioners, treat the total person, not just the condition. Ernie says this best:

> This means to take into account every individual. We look at the individual person and treat the patients according to their capabilities. We have to be able to motivate and enable the patient to participate in [his or her] treatment plan. We often require a little more patience in dealing with the older person...everything should be individualized, and we should be able to innovate our treatment plans to suit [him or her].

When seeing your physiotherapist for the first time, you will be required to answer some questions regarding your neck pain and your overall state of health. You will also be asked to fill out a health questionnaire and list your prescribed medications. You should inform your therapist if there are any questions you do not understand; he will guide you through the process.

Your therapist may also request current X-ray results and any other information he may deem important. Because the results of early trauma are often played out in our bodies when we are older, he will be particularly interested in any falls or any other trauma you may have suffered throughout your life, as well as your previous occupations. You will then undergo an in-depth examination of your posture, range of motion, and muscle strength. Your therapist will also conduct tests of your sensation, reflexes, and stability of the joints in your neck. The examination will include similar tests of your upper limbs. A thorough examination is especially important for older adults because as Ernie explains:

> Older patients often have pre-existing conditions and more severe postural changes. They may also have a loss of strength in general. Other medical issues can include cardiovascular or neurological conditions, diabetes, and metabolic issues. Further, the medications that [older adults] take to manage those conditions may make their physical treatment a little more challenging as they may not be able to concentrate normally and find it difficult to follow instructions.

Other age-related issues must be taken into consideration when one is receiving physiotherapy treatments. Problems with balance, poor eyesight or poor hearing, and language barriers can make treatment more challenging. Memory impairment or problems with one's ability to concentrate also present as problematic. Therefore, in treating the older person, it is often necessary to involve family, extended family, or friends in the treatment protocol. Encouragement from family members can be very supportive for an older person. When your physiotherapist is dedicated to working with you rather than simply your condition, he will always find an innovative way to provide treatment.

Some examples of treatments your physiotherapist may suggest include pain relief, range of motion and strengthening exercises, specific mobilization of the joints in the neck, and education regarding your condition and your treatment plan. In addition, your physiotherapist will want to know about how you manage your activities of daily living (ADL). Other specific techniques that may be offered are mechanical traction and electrotherapy. All patients will receive a home-exercise program involving the neck and the upper back.

Partnering with Your Physiotherapist

There are few things more rewarding than working with a health-care provider to improve your overall heath and sense of well-being, especially when the reduction of pain and discomfort is the shared goal. But it is important to remember that physiotherapy is largely an active treatment approach rather than a passive one like massage or reflexology. Expect homework and know that compliance is a must.

As we age, compliance may become more demanding due to other health challenges. We may need someone to remind us to perform the prescribed exercise regimen at home. We may also need an observer to ensure that we're doing the exercises in a way that is beneficial rather than detrimental to recovery. Again, the involvement of family and friends is emphasized.

Two of the most important activities that you can undertake between visits are to walk and practice good posture. Another activity to help build strength and improve balance is water exercise. Ernie underscores that you "don't need to swim to gain benefit. You can wear flotation devices and move, which is really pleasant. You can walk in water, for example, which is more comfortable for patients with severe hip, ankle, or knee problems and even back problems."

No matter the physical activity you choose, one important piece of advice for people with osteoarthritis is that body movement is essential. "One thing we know," Ernie emphasizes, "is that the more active we are even in a gentle way, the better our outcomes will be."

Physiotherapists recommend that clients avoid recreational activities that require reaching and/or a head-forward or a craning position. For example, golf, bowling, tennis, and weight lifting can all prove detrimental when one is suffering from acute or sub-acute neck or upper back pain. Even the more sedentary recreational activities, such as card and board games, knitting, crocheting, and extended work at a computer, can prove detrimental. Playing musical instruments such as the piano, violin, or cello may also be problematic. Therefore, anyone participating in such activities must remember to get up and move around occasionally or stretch.

Despite neck problems, adults derive pleasure from the independence they experience when driving. However, Ernie cautions, "if one has an inability to check traffic by turning his or her head from side to side, he or she should be prepared to give up driving until his or her condition has improved."

Ways to Manage a Painful Episode

Neck pain ebbs and flows in duration, intensity, and frequency. It can be acute, sub-acute, or chronic in nature, or become acute within a chronic pain syndrome. Ernie has an approach to treating neck pain that gives consideration to the characteristics of each client's description of his or her pain experience. You may find his following plan of care helpful.

Acute Stage (0 to 4-6 days)

In addition to medication, the application of ice is an excellent pain-reduction strategy. If your pain level is severe, apply an ice pack for fifteen to twenty minutes at a time with a lapse of three to four hours in between as needed during waking hours. You can do this for forty-eight to seventy-two hours. You can also use a soft collar during this phase, but it is not usually recommended for more than a three-to five-day period, as the muscles will weaken and the range of motion will decrease. If you have pain at night, you may use a soft collar to aid sleep.

Sub-acute Stage (4 to 6-10 days)

When your pain has subsided, you can try heat for the same time periods to find relief. If using a beanbag for heat or cold, you should always use it while sitting in a recliner or lying in bed so that you avoid straining your neck with the weight. During this stage, you may begin postural and range-of-motion exercises, gentle manual therapy, and stretching.

Chronic Stage (10 days and onward)

During the chronic state, you would normally continue with the exercises previously prescribed by your physiotherapist and include strengthening exercises, traction, and manual therapy. Other complementary therapies can also help you to have success with physiotherapy. For example, acupuncture, acupressure, hypnotherapy, reflexology, and massage can be useful. They improve blood flow, reduce pain, and encourage relaxation, all of which will help you to feel better and increase your willingness to move more. Remember that movement is essential for the body. Bodies, joints, and muscles are all meant to move.

There are other simple steps you can take to find comfort. Ernie suggests two. The first recommends a change in the number of pillows used at night. He notes that many people use more than one pillow when sleeping. If you take a minute and visualize what two or more pillows do to your head and neck, you can envision how your head and neck are pushed forward in frontal and side flexion. Imagine what eight hours of that position is doing to your neck and your pain experience. Ernie advises one pillow; no pillow is better if you can manage without one.

Ernie's second suggestion involves ergonomics; a related science that complements physiotherapy. Ergonomics focuses on making daily living and working easier while protecting your body from the long-term consequences of poor posture and degeneration. Good ergonomics can also help a person move through a painful stage to once again enjoy activities of daily life. Simply stated, ergonomics is a science that aims to make environments more comfortable and efficient for those living, working, and playing within them. For example, sound ergonomic principles can help one determine where to place appliances and utensils so that they are within easy and comfortable reach, eliminating the need for craning, reaching, and head-forward positions.

For someone who is short, standing on a small, safe stool while working at a countertop may prove useful. Ironing can often be accomplished from a seated position. Washing machines and dryers can be placed on platforms to make loading and unloading easier. Look around your home and determine how changes in your environment can make daily life more comfortable. Consultation with your physiotherapist, occupational therapist, or other professionals with special training in ergonomics can make a huge difference in how you manage your environment and live a pain-free life.

Conclusion

Physiotherapists are health-care professionals highly educated in the anatomy and physiology of the human body. Physiotherapists are interested in body movement, function, stability and balance, and the maintenance and restoration of the entire musculoskeletal system. They use clinical evidence, diagnostic tests, clinical examination, and the client's description of the pain experience to plan and direct an appropriate course of care and treatment.

Cognizant of the individual as unique, physiotherapists provide individualized care and treatment to the total person. In this way, they are teachers as well as healers. Their ability to help clients self-manage neck pain places them in high demand as health-care providers.

PART THREE: Putting it all Together

Introduction

The complementary practitioners presented in the pages of this book have provided many important lessons. While each practice is different, there are still common threads within the lessons. We have gathered those threads together to create a tapestry of wisdom from which you can select the strands most relevant to you.

Taking a holistic approach is not about going to one therapist or another; it is about transforming your approach to caring for yourself. Included in the approach is the acceptance of both complementary therapies and traditional allopathic medicine as the route to healing. Holistic medicine is also about your capacity for and willingness to change your way of thinking, choosing, and acting in support of healing your body, mind, and spirit. As you reflect on these common threads, it will be helpful to ask yourself the following questions and record your responses in your journal. Before you begin, read over all the questions and the review of the core lessons.

Journal Work

> a. Is the information presented new? If so, in what way does it impact my lifestyle?
>
> b. What will I need to change?
>
> c. Am I willing to invest my energy in the work of becoming well?
>
> d. Do I have the energy and support I will need to embark on a healing journey?
>
> e. If not, am I willing to continue with the pain I am currently experiencing?

Lesson: Understand Holistic Practice

Each complementary practitioner interviewed had a therapeutic understanding of the root cause(s) of chronic neck pain, and without exception those causes arose from the multifaceted and complex nature of each individual client. Holistic practice means that the therapist takes into account the cognitive, emotional, physical, social, environmental, and spiritual aspects of each person.

Because of the complex nature of human beings, it is sometimes necessary to engage additional practitioners in the overall treatment plan. When complementary health practitioners work together with medical doctors, social workers, and other complementary therapists, they are working collaboratively. As such, the term *complementary* is being replaced by *collaborative/ integrative*. In a collaborative/integrative model, the client is offered a wider range of treatment options informed by medical, pharmaceutical, and complementary practices.

Embedded in the notion of teams comprised of health-care providers is the acceptance of you, the client, as the center and creator of your team. When you see yourself as the creator and in the center, your team becomes not only client-centered but also client-directed. You and your family/extended family become the unit of care and service. It is an important distinction because rather than something that is done *to* you, your care is performed *with* you in a partnership different from previous provider-patient relationships.

A partnership suggests equality, which means that no treatment can be undertaken without your informed consent. Informed consent means that health-care practitioners provide you with whatever information you may require or request in a way that is clear and acceptable to you. Particularly as we age, we may need that information presented with patience, understanding, and a willingness to answer all questions at the time they are asked. Having material in writing for frequent review and providing diagrams are two useful ways your practitioner can clarify information. You should feel comfortable requesting that written and/or graphic information be made available to you if you believe it will help.

Many of the practitioners we interviewed spoke of the importance of fully hearing the voice of their client. Active listening is one of the most respectful gifts that health-care providers can give. You are the person on your journey toward lifestyle change. The job of the professional is to help you accomplish your goal, and that will be nearly impossible if your practitioner isn't listening to you. Not all of us are the same, so if you feel unheard or if you believe that the two of you are not a good match, be brave and seek a change to a practitioner with whom you feel connected.

Lesson: You Have Choice

A partnership means that you also have responsibilities to fulfill. If you decide to enlist a complementary practitioner, you must be ready to make the changes and do the work that will relieve your neck pain and return you to your quality of life. What does it mean to be ready?

Readiness implies an open mind—your willingness to follow recommendations or approaches that may be foreign to you. Willingness means you hold a curiosity about the array of possibilities presented and adopt an attitude of trust that a solution can be found. Most of us have visited medical practitioners many times. We have come to expect a certain way of being examined and treated for what ails us. The tools and techniques of complementary practitioners may seem alien at first, so your job is to remain open and willing to participate.

Participation means that you listen, ask questions, and involve yourself in treatment decisions. Participation also means that you take responsibility for completing homework such as doing an exercise routine, making changes in food choices, or adding vitamins, herbs, or nutritional supplements to your daily routine.

When you become an active participant in your wellness choices, you realize that you know your body best and that your healthy choices make a difference. Through having the underlying causes of your condition explained, you begin to understand that you can change many of your pain-inducing behaviors and move yourself toward improved health and well-being. Keep in mind that the goal of health-care practitioners is to move you into *self*-management through education and open discussion.

Self-management of your neck pain means that you have grown in self-awareness, self-confidence, and self-empowerment. Knowing how to monitor your own condition and what choices you can make to keep your improvements on track is empowering. Self-management helps you in social situations, too, because when pain is relieved and confidence restored, you are more inclined to become engaged in life. The quality of your life is restored. Self-management enlivens your spirit. As you grow in the awareness that you are a multifaceted individual, unique in the universe, you begin to truly appreciate a collaborative approach. So make it your intention to participate with your complementary therapist and trust in his or her ability to help you heal with confidence.

Lesson: Each Person's Pain Experience is Unique

Many people think of pain as an indicator that something is wrong with their physical body. In this way, pain is an important signal that one's physical body needs attention. When pain is acute, our first thoughts involve immediate relief. Unwanted pain or discomfort is the symptom that sends us to the emergency room or to our physicians for help. Generally, acute pain can be relieved quickly through the use of drugs, usually narcotics for severe pain. When the source of pain is identified and treatment provided, the underlying process creating the pain is eliminated.

However, when pain is chronic, it is a total-person experience that affects every aspect of daily living and overall quality of life. Pain can be all engulfing, making it difficult to remember when the pain first began and even harder to be convinced that it can ever be completely relieved. For some people the pain may never be fully relieved, but it can be managed and reduced to a point where one can live with it and still enjoy life. Learning how to manage your pain is an important goal of collaborative health strategies.

Long-term pain impacts us cognitively in that it can interfere with memory. In the elderly, pain can impair a person's memory and induce mental confusion. Memory impairment and confusion in the elderly can be misdiagnosed as the onset of dementia, and such an assumption can in turn create fear and anxiety, further increasing one's pain.

Pain can also be exhausting, reducing an individual's desire to be involved in family gatherings and other social activities. Pain can interfere with eating, exercising, and sleeping, and that produces other serious health challenges in older people. When a person is in constant pain, she may withdraw from social contact and then experience the suffering that comes from loneliness and isolation. Older people often fear pain at the end of their lives more than they fear death itself. As we age, pain becomes a serious consideration, and being pain-free becomes a resource for daily living.

We learned from Dr. Saunderson that the brain and the body are inseparable and in constant communication. The way in which the mind can affect the body during times of intense relaxation grows more profound as we age. Because older adults bring more experience and wisdom, they generally find it easier to move into a state of calm and let go. In a state of calm, the mind can change, or reframe the experience of the body; that is, the mind can interrupt the pain signal from the brain and change the intensity of the pain experience. With guidance from a qualified therapeutic hypnotherapist, self-hypnosis can become part of a person's pain-management routine.

Lesson: Understand the Cause(s) of Your Neck Pain

Knowing the root causes of pain and the ways to address those root causes is perhaps a more familiar way to manage pain. Therefore, we asked each of the complementary practitioners how they understand the causes of neck pain and soreness in older persons. Most of the practitioners interviewed shared a common understanding of the multiple underlying causes of neck pain, especially as their clients grow older. These causes include trauma, poor posture, metabolic changes, poor nutrition, blocked energy, emotions, self-image, stress and challenging relationships.

Trauma

Most practitioners agree that neck problems in the elderly began much earlier in life, usually stemming from a physical injury such as a fall, motor vehicle accident, or sports injury. Sometimes the injury occurred so long ago that it was lost from memory; other times, the injury played a more recent role in developing a chronic pain syndrome. Like uncorrected posture, over the long term, changes in the spine negatively affect quality of life as one grows older.

Poor Posture

There are a number of environmental conditions that contribute to poor posture and subsequent neck pain. For example, people whose work life involved desk work, sewing, carpentry, and other occupations that required them to hold their heads down for an extended period will likely encounter neck problems with age. Others whose work required heavy lifting and carrying will also be at risk for joint, muscle, and bone difficulties. Caregiving for a spouse or child who is physically challenged can, over time, take its toll on one's physical health, as can occupations that are defined by bending, lifting, and pulling.

Heredity and habit can play into poor posture. We tend to walk, sit and stand like our parents. If their habit is one of rounded shoulders, hip forward stance, there is a probability that we'll mimic that posture. Postural protection of a weakened or injured area can also create a habit that persists after the injury is healed or weakness is eliminated.

Some older people have a staccato way of walking due to their tendency to shuffle their feet as they walk. Uneven surfaces or surfaces that are carpeted make this posture unsafe due to the high probability of a fall.

Inappropriate footwear can cause misalignment of the spinal column and tax one's musculoskeletal frame. Any woman who has attempted to wear stilettos heels during a number of hours standing and/or walking can attest to the discomfort of shoes designed for fashion rather than comfort.

Metabolic Changes

Normal processes of aging such as pre- and postmenopausal changes in hormone levels that may produce weight gain and depression can contribute to neck pain. Emotional fluctuations represent changes in body chemistry. Imbalances in an individual's body chemistry both cause and affect one's pain experience. Poor nutritional choices and liver and digestive problems can also contribute to weight gain and other serious metabolic changes that in turn lead to chronic pain. Loss of trace minerals and calcium is a precursor to osteoporosis and can account for changes in bone structure and neck pain. Food choices also affect metabolism and can intensify the experience of pain. Some foods are thought to actually cause inflammation while others feed it. Working with a doctor of natural or Chinese medicine can help you improve your knowledge of specific dietary changes that can lead to pain reduction and/or elimination.

Poor Nutrition: Dietary Deficiencies

Food is our fuel, and nutritional foods are converted into energy. Non-nutritional foods such as processed foods are converted into toxins that create and perpetuate inflammation. These are known as pro-inflammation foods. Reducing and/or eliminating them from your diet will prove beneficial. They include but are not limited to the following categories of foods:

- sugar-sweetened beverages, pastries, desserts, candy, and snacks
- vegetable cooking oils that contain high amounts of omega-6 fatty acids
- trans fats: deep-fried food, fast food, hydrogenated vegetable oil, and vegetable shortening
- refined grains: white flour, white rice, white pasta, boxed cereals

Partnering with an integrated nutritional counselor will help you change your poor dietary habits to those that are higher in nutrients and beneficial to pain management.

Blocked Energy

The body is a living bioenergetic system that transforms the flow of energy through the body. Living systems like our bodies depend on the transfer of energy internally and externally. When the body's energy is blocked, pain, dysfunction, and disease can develop. Doctors of Chinese medicine, acupuncturists, and reflexologists all work to unblock the body's energy channels so that energy can continue to flow uninterrupted.

Emotions

Pain is also an emotional experience. Daily stress causes our muscles to contract and tighten, producing pain in the neck and shoulders as well as pain that radiates to our head and can cause severe headaches. Long-term low-grade stress can be even more damaging because tension tends to be happening below our awareness. Over time, even when we feel relaxed, our muscles retain the memory of stress and strain, resulting in a chronic pain pattern.

Self-Image

Negative changes in our physical appearance, our body image, and our ability to work as hard or as long can lead to depression, overeating, and weight gain, all of which taxes an aging spine. Long-standing pain itself may have led to despair, which contributes to the circle of pain.

Women tend to be more emotionally upset by pain than men. Women, as caregivers, may be uncomfortable with having to be cared for rather than giving care. Such a perceived loss of power can be an affront to one's self-image and bring a sense of victimization. Men tend to manage pain more stoically but may not be able to manage the same intensity of pain.

Stress and Challenging Relationships

Real-time stressors such as financial worries, difficult family relationships, or a declining social network through the loss of family and friends can induce or exacerbate pain. Avoidance of difficult relationships because of a reluctance to speak up can also lead to pain. Often, older people believe that they have no voice. As they begin to slow down, the world seems to pass them by. Family members, professional caregivers and significant others may insist that they know best for an aging parent or client. Feeling unheard and pushed into the background can lead to passivity, especially if one feels and believes that she has been left behind by family, friends, and other care providers. Human beings have a need to be heard and to belong. Finding one person—a pastor, a spiritual advisor, a professional counselor—to talk over problems with is beneficial no matter one's age.

Learning to be more self-assertive can free you to live more independently. Self-assertiveness can improve your relationships and decrease stress. However, being more assertive is difficult for someone used to being passive or afraid to speak up. Many communities offer self-improvement programs, so check your local newspaper for courses in assertiveness training. Often you can speak with an instructor prior to the beginning of a training program to determine whether the training is right for you.

Lesson: Pain Can Be Relieved

We learned about some major physical causes of pain and some emotional contributing factors—the inside and the outside causes. One can clearly see the mind-body connection at work—what we believe, we feel; and what we feel, we believe. Now we can use the inside and outside as a way to approach pain relief.

There is a simple truth about chronic neck pain. When one views pain from the perspective of a total-person experience, it's clear that drugs alone cannot relieve the physical, emotional, social, cognitive, and spiritual suffering that accompanies chronic pain. We have researched and developed the lessons for pain relief around a holistic approach. Although we have placed the aspects of pain relief into separate categories, because they are interconnected, they all overlap and intertwine. Therefore, suggestions and recommendations in one area may be useful in another and are presented in point form. Remember that these are only suggestions; you should always follow a plan of treatment that feels right for you and complements who you are.

Physical Pain Relief: Medication

- Always ensure that you have a complete medical examination by your physician to determine the underlying cause of pain.
- Take medication as directed by your physician, and take it consistently so the pain does not get ahead of the medication's ability to relieve it.

Physical Pain Relief: Posture Awareness

- Become mindful of your posture.
- Walk consciously with your head in an upright position instead of stooping.
- Avoid shuffling your feet while walking. Use heel-toe imagery so that you are stepping consciously.
- Use handrails (if available) instead of looking down at each step when you descend stairs.
- Hobbies such as needlework, crossword or jigsaw puzzles, carving, and weaving should be undertaken for short periods of time with rest and gentle neck stretches between

sessions. Be mindful to use appropriate table heights to avoid bending your head down more than necessary.

- Sleep on a good-quality mattress and use as flat a pillow as you can to maintain good sleeping posture.

- Consider asking for help from a professional trained in ergonomics.

Physical Pain Relief: Exercise

- Try something new like yoga, pilates, or qigong for exercise.

- Remember that any movement, even gentle movement, is exercise.

- Consider other complementary therapies for pain relief as outlined in the book.

Physical Pain Relief: Diet

- Eat four to five small meals a day.

- Increase your intake of fruits, vegetables, and whole foods.

- Eat at least five servings of colorful vegetables, including a good amount of greens each day.

- Avoid artificially sweetened foods and drinks.

- Restrict your intake of red meat, and increase your intake of organic chicken, wild fish, and legumes.

- Consume at least eight glasses of water or other liquids like green or herbals teas daily, but avoid sugar-sweetened drinks and excessive coffee.

- Purchase organic and locally grown foods when possible.
- Check with your physician, integrative health counselor, naturopath, or doctor of Chinese medicine to see whether you have specific nutritional deficiencies such as calcium, vitamins (especially D), omega-3, or other trace minerals.

Emotional Pain Relief

- Avoid withdrawing into yourself.
- If you feel that you are slipping into depression, phone a friend or family member.
- Be willing to talk things over with a trusted friend. Seek out a counselor (a paid friend) if you believe that there is no other person with whom you wish to talk. Having a listener is very important in helping you to stay the course and reach your health goals more easily.
- Recognize that everyone ages and undergoes natural physical and emotional changes. Keep yourself well-groomed and active. Exercise is a good way to boost your mood.
- Consider clinical hypnotherapy to help release old wounds and manage stress.

Social Pain Relief

- Avoid isolating yourself.
- Keep physically active—join an exercise, quilting, card-playing, or music group.

- Contact family and friends often. Join in family celebrations.
- Join a senior center. Get involved with the activities offered. Go on trips and outings.
- Mentor a child or teenager. There is a demand for literacy volunteers and for foster grandparenting programs so you can share your time, love, and experience.

Cognitive Pain Relief (Keeping Your Mind Active)

- Read or listen to audiobooks.
- Discuss current events with family and friends.
- Attend a lecture at your local community college or church.
- Play games that require strategy. Do crossword puzzles or Sudoku.
- Learn a new hobby or a new language.

Spiritual Pain Relief

- All of the above activities feed the spirit. Additional activities include the following:
- Each day as you arise, set an intention for what you would like to do with your day. Include with whom you would like to share your day and how you can sow love in your world.
- Practice gratitude.

- Forgive.
- Practice silence and prayer.
- Join with your faith community to worship.
- Seek out a spiritual advisor.
- Volunteer with your church, synagogue, or temple, and work on behalf of others who are having life difficulties.
- Create items for the church bazaar.
- Donate to a family in a developing country; sponsor a child.
- Read inspirational literature.

The above lists offer only a few suggestions provided to help you engage in your life. As you can see, there are many ways to manage your pain and discomfort. If you accept that you are capable of a pain-free life, you can adopt some of the methods mentioned or you can seek the help and guidance of a complementary healthcare provider. Either way, the ultimate goal for you is to be skilled at managing your pain, not to have the pain manage you.

If you have found some comfort in the pages that have been offered, we've done our job. Now is the time to do yours. We know that with an open mind, a grateful heart, and informed choice, you can find your way to comfort and healing. It is our greatest wish for you.

For more information please visit us at http://www.therapiesforneckpain.com

INDEX

Laraine Crampton, LAc, BS Ed, MPW, MLA, MATCM

Licensed Acupuncturist (LAc)
Bachelor of Science in Secondary Education (BSc Ed)
Master of Professional Writing (MPW)
Master of Liberal Arts (MLA)
Master of Acupuncture and Traditional Chinese Medicine (MATCM)

David Wu, DC

Doctor of Chiropractic (DC)
Certified Alphabioticist
Qualified Medical Evaluator
Industrial Disability Examiner
Certified Bio Cranial Therapist

Maria Redinger, LAc, MATCM, Dipl. O. M., CMT, CST

Licensed Acupuncturist (LAc)
Master of Acupuncture and Traditional Chinese Medicine (MATCM)

Diplomate of Oriental Medicine (Dipl. O.M.)
Certified Massage Therapist (CMT)
CranioSacral Therapist courses through the Upledger Institute (CST)

Linda Henderson, DNM, DCT, DTCM, H.D., RBT, ROHP, RM

Doctor of Natural Medicine (DNM)
Doctor of Clinical Therapies (pastoral) (DCT)
Doctor of Traditional Chinese Medicine (DTCM)
Doctor of Homeopathy (H.D.)
Registered Biofeedback Therapist (RBT)
Registered Orthomolecular Health Practitioner (ROHP) and Reiki Master (RM)

Jack A. Marriott, CMR, CRI, CBS, CBI, MR, CSM

Certified Master Reflexologist (CMR)
Certified Reflexology Instructor (CRI)
Certified Biofeedback Specialist (CBS)
Certified Biofeedback Instructor (CBI)
Master Reflexologist (MR)
Certified Shopping Centre Manager (CSM) International Council of Shopping Centres (ICSC)

Dr. V. R. Brick Saunderson, D. Min, RCCH, CHtA, CMC

Doctor of Ministry (D. Min)
Registered Clinical Counselling Hypnotherapist (RCCH)
Certified Hypno-anesthesia and Pain Management Therapist (CHtA)
Certified Mastery Coach (CMC)

Mona E. Saunderson, RPC, RCCH, CHtA

Registered Professional Counsellor (RPC)
Registered Clinical Counselling Hypnotherapist (RCCH)
Certified Hypno-anesthesia and Pain Management Therapist (CHtA)

Patrick A. Martin, Jr., BA, AAS, HC, MA Candidate
Bachelor of Arts (BA) Integrative Health and Humanities

Associate of Applied Science Human Services (AAS)
Health Counselor (HC)
Masters of Arts, Psychology (MA Candidate), LIOS College, Saybrook University

Erica Trokey, DC, BSc, CPI

Doctorate of Chiropractic (DC)
Bachelor of Science (BSc) Human Biology
Certified Reformer and Mat Pilates, Balanced Body® University (CPI)

Ernest Ball, BSc.PT, MCPA

Bachelor of Science, Physiotherapy (BSc PT)
Member Canadian Physiotherapy Association (MCPA)

JOURNAL WORK

Journaling or expressive writing is a simple, gentle and inexpensive healing technique. I consider it a powerful therapeutic tool to learn more about yourself and become aware of how your mind and emotions can influence you physically.

Andrew Weil, MD

My Journal

Manufactured by Amazon.ca
Bolton, ON

11100795R00099